WITHDRAWN
WRIGHT STATE UNIVERSITY LIBRARIES

Management of Migraine

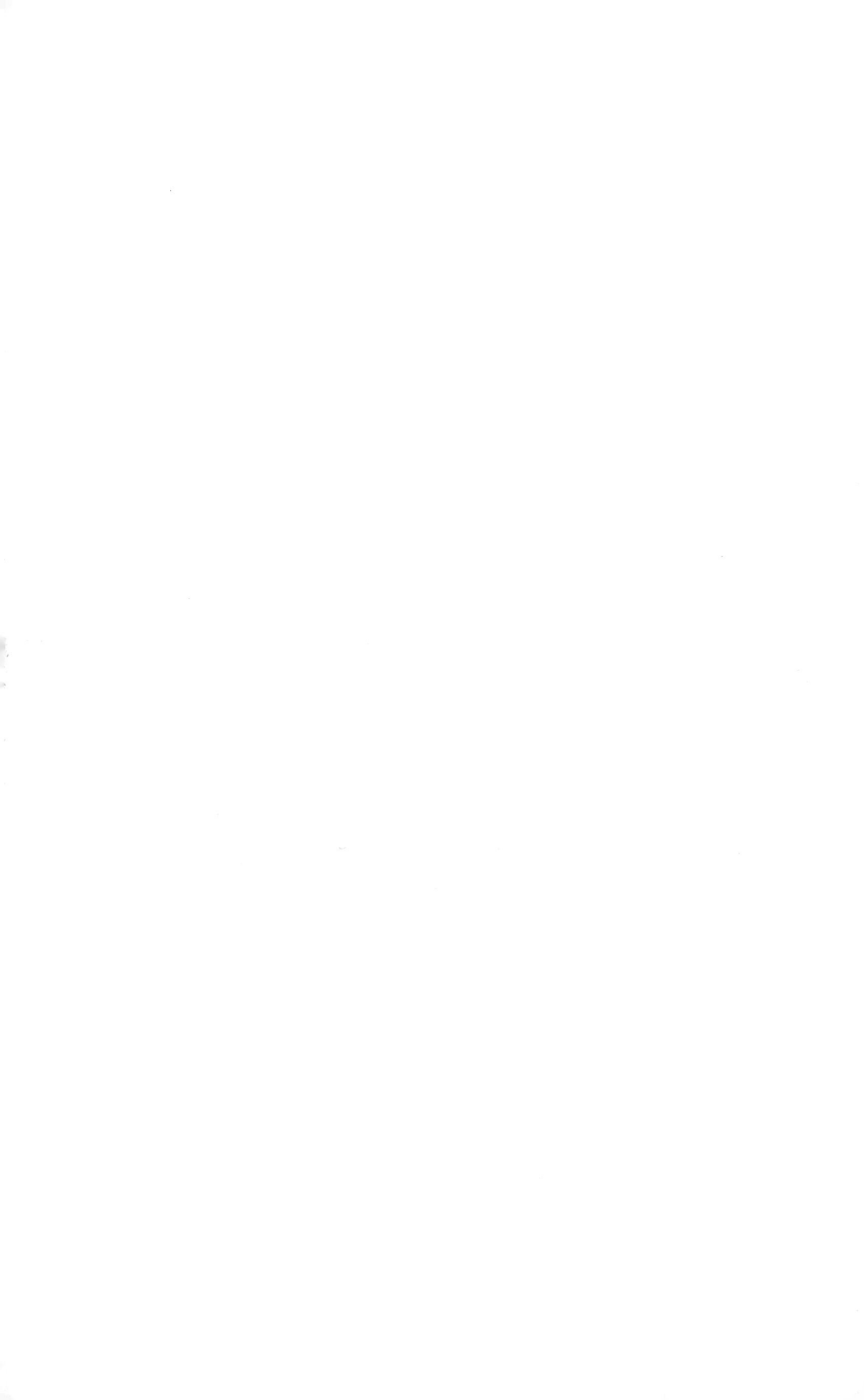

Management of Migraine

Egilius L.H. Spierings, M.D., Ph.D.

Physician in Neurology and Director of Headache Research, Brigham and Women's Hospital; Lecturer in Neurology, Harvard Medical School, Boston

Butterworth-Heinemann
Boston Oxford Melbourne Singapore Toronto Munich New Delhi Tokyo

WL
344
S755
1996

Copyright © 1996 by Butterworth-Heinemann

 A member of the Reed Elsevier group

All rights reserved.

No part of this publication may be reproduced, stored in a retrieval system, or transmitted in any form or by any means, electronic, mechanical, photocopying, recording, or otherwise, without the prior written permission of the publisher.

Every effort has been made to ensure that the drug dosage schedules within this text are accurate and conform to standards accepted at time of publication. However, as treatment recommendations vary in the light of continuing research and clinical experience, the reader is advised to verify drug dosage schedules herein with information found on product information sheets. This is especially true in cases of new or infrequently used drugs.

 Recognizing the importance of preserving what has been written, Butterworth-Heinemann prints its books on acid-free paper whenever possible.

Library of Congress Cataloging-in-Publication Data

Spierings, Egilius L. H., 1953-
   Management of migraine / Egilius L. H. Spierings.
      p.   cm.
   Includes bibliographical references and index.
   ISBN 0-7506-9623-0 (alk. paper)
   1. Migraine. I. Title.
   [DNLM: 1. Migraine—drug therapy. 2. Migraine WL 344 S755m 1996]
   RC392.S64   1996
   616.8'57—dc20
   DNLM/DLC
   for Library of Congress   95-31182
                                                                         CIP

British Library Cataloguing-in-Publication Data
A catalogue record for this book is available from the British Library.

The publisher offers discounts on bulk orders of this book.
For information, please write:
Manager of Special Sales
Butterworth-Heinemann
313 Washington Street
Newton, MA 021581626

10 9 8 7 6 5 4 3 2 1

Printed in the United States of America

Dedicated to my son, Sven

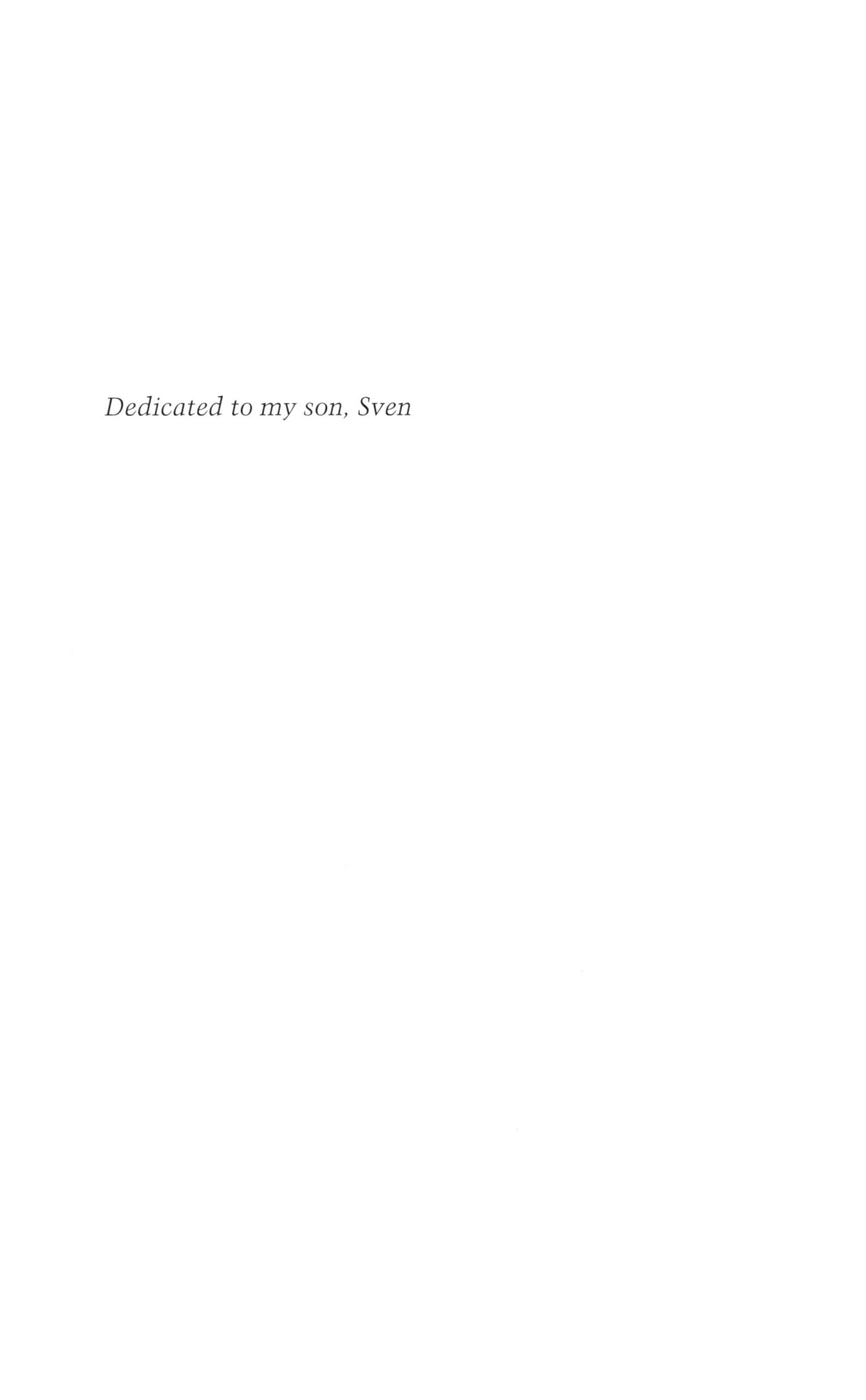

Contents

Preface ... ix

1. Definition and Classification ... 1
2. Symptomatology and Pathogenesis ... 7
3. Diagnosis and Differential Diagnosis ... 21
4. Abortive Pharmacological Treatment ... 27
5. Preventive Pharmacological Treatment ... 65
6. Endogenous and Exogenous Trigger Factors ... 105
7. Headache and Migraine in Childhood ... 119
8. Cluster Headache and Paroxysmal Hemicrania ... 131

Index ... 143

Preface

This book is about migraine, one of the most common painful conditions of mankind, known to us through writings since as early as 3,000 BC. It is a condition that causes disability, be it often temporary, and strains the personal and professional development. Nevertheless, little is known about it in scientific terms and, hence, its treatment is mostly empirical. The treatment of migraine is the focus of this book, discussed on the basis of available studies against the background of extensive personal experience.

On the basis of a review of many studies, the prevalence of migraine in the general population is estimated at 9 percent in men and 16 percent in women.[1] The prevalence of migraine increases rapidly during the first and second decades of life, remains at the same level until the fourth or fifth decade, then declines slowly but steadily with the advancement in age. A recent study of a sample of the Danish population revealed a one-year prevalence of migraine of 6 percent in men and 15 percent in women.[2] In the United States, a sample of the population was surveyed in a study that considered only severe headaches. It revealed a one-year prevalence of migraine of 6 percent in men and 18 percent in women.[3] In this study, it was found also that the one-year prevalence of migraine is the highest in both men and women between the ages of 35 and 45. In addition, the one-year prevalence of migraine was found to be associated strongly with (household) income (i.e., in the lowest income group—less than $10,000—it is more than 60 percent higher than in the two highest income groups—the same as or greater than $30,000). No differences in one-year prevalence were found between the white and black races, urban and rural residence, and regions of residence in the United States.

Many of those who have migraine never seek medical consultation. Migraine is often present in the family and, therefore, the patient is familiar with the condition and knows that its prognosis is *medically* benign. With regard to the potential of obtaining relief, there is generally the implicit understanding that there is no cure. However, there also seems to be the belief that the medical profession cannot do anything for the patient that the patient cannot do privately. The above-mentioned population study conducted in the United States underscores the extent to which migraine is underdiagnosed and undertreated. Among other things, it was found that 71 percent of men and 59 percent of women with migraine in the general population are never diagnosed by a physician.[4] This despite the fact that all these people have severe headaches and 80 percent of them experiences at least some degree of disability with their headaches. The symptoms most strongly associated with a physician-diagnosis of migraine are vomiting, blurred vision, and visual or sensory aura. A physician-diagnosis of migraine is also less likely if the annual household income is $10,000 or less.

With regard to medication intake, it was found that most patients with migraine, that is, 67 percent of men and 57 percent of women, use nonprescription medications to treat their headaches.[5] Only 28 percent of men and 40 percent of women take prescription medications, and 5 percent of men and 3 percent of women take no medications at all. The highest use of prescription medications was found in the patients who experience vomiting or visual aura with their headaches, symptoms also associated with physician-diagnosis. The use of prescription medications was also found to be related to the frequency and duration of the headaches and to the disability caused by them.

References

1. Goldstein M, Chen TC. The epidemiology of disabling headache. Adv Neurol 1982; 33:37–390.
2. Rasmussen BK, Jensen R, Schroll M, Olesen J. Epidemiology of headache in a general population-A prevalence study. J Clin Epidemiol 1991; 44:1147–1157.
3. Stewart WF, Lipton RB, Celentano DD, Reed ML. Prevalence of migraine headache in the United States. JAMA 1992; 267:64–69.
4. Lipton RB, Stewart WF, Celentano DD, Reed ML. Undiagnosed migraine headaches: A comparison of symptom-based and reported physician diagnosis. Arch Intern Med 1992; 152:1273–1278.
5. Celentano DD, Stewart WF, Lipton RB, Reed ML. Medication use and disability among migraineurs: A national probability sample survey. Headache 1992; 32:223–228.

CHAPTER 1

Definition and Classification

Definition

Migraine is a paroxysmal disorder with relative freedom from symptoms between attacks. The attacks consist of transient focal neurological symptoms and/or headache. The transient focal neurological symptoms are almost always sensory in nature, generally visual, and sometimes somatosensory. However, the headache is usually so intense that it interferes with the ability to function. Also, it is generally so intense that it is associated with such other symptoms as light and noise sensitivity, nausea, and vomiting. These symptoms usually follow the onset of the headache and increase in intensity as the headache progresses. The transient focal neurological symptoms, on the other hand, almost always precede the onset of the headache or occur during its initial phase. These symptoms are often referred to as *aura symptoms* (the term that will be employed throughout this text).

The attacks of migraine generally last less than one hour when they merely consist of transient focal neurological symptoms but last from hours to days when headache is present. When the transient focal neurological symptoms occur without headache, the condition is referred to as *isolated migraine aura* or *migraine aura without headache.* When both the transient focal neurological symptoms and headache occur, the condition is referred to as *classic migraine* or *migraine with aura.* When the headache occurs by itself, the condition is referred to as *common migraine* or *migraine without aura.*

As with many (if not most) medical conditions, migraine possesses a hereditary component. This component manifests itself in a positive family history (i.e., the occurrence of migraine in first-degree relatives) in 60 to 70 percent of patients. In addition, it is estimated that the risk of developing migraine is 45 percent when one parent has migraine and 70 percent when both parents are affected. The onset of migraine almost always occurs within the first three decades of life, often in the teenage or adolescent years.

Unfortunately for many of those affected, migraine is a lifelong condition, although the headaches very often abate with the advancement of age.

The frequency with which the attacks occur varies tremendously and can be as low as once per year or as high as once or twice per week. The frequency of the attacks varies not only between individuals but also between periods of time within the same individual. The variation in frequency of the attacks is related to the sensitivity of migraine to many endogenous and exogenous factors, often referred to as *trigger factors*. One important endogenous trigger factor is the estrogen cycle in women, which largely accounts for two or three times greater prevalence of migraine in women than in men.

Spectrum of vascular headaches

Migraine can be considered at the end of a spectrum of vascular headaches (Figure 1.1). It is surpassed by tension-type (muscle-contraction) vascular headache, which, however, is not a purely vascular headache condition. The spectrum of vascular headaches starts with *jabs and jolts,* sharp headache pains which last seconds.[1] These headache pains occur by themselves, as in the jabs-and-jolts syndrome, or in association with other vascular headaches, such as migraine or cluster headache. *Paroxysmal hemicrania* are unilateral headaches which last from 10 to 30 minutes and occur 5 to 15 times per day.[2] *Cluster headache* are also unilateral headaches but their duration is longer, and they last from 30 minutes to 2 hours. The headaches in cluster headache also occur less frequently, usually once or twice per day. The vascular headaches respond abortively *and* preventively to vasoconstrictor medications. The shorter-lasting vascular headaches (i.e., jabs and jolts and paroxysmal hemicrania) also respond preventively to indomethacin (Indocid, UK; Indocin, US).

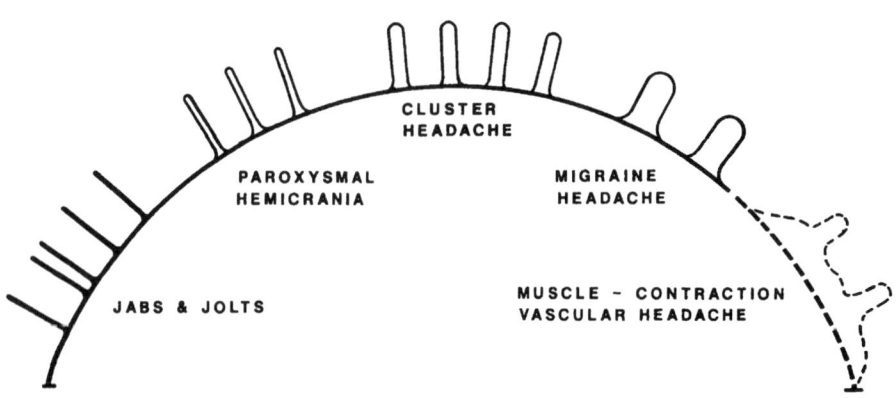

FIGURE 1.1 The spectrum of vascular headaches, including jabs and jolts, paroxysmal hemicrania, cluster headache, and migraine.

Classification

In the headache classification as proposed in 1962 by the National Institute of Neurological Diseases and Blindness (NINDB), migraine is classified under the category of vascular headaches of the migraine type.[3] This category includes classic migraine, common migraine, cluster headache, hemiplegic and ophthalmoplegic migraine, and lower-half headache (facial migraine). These headache conditions are thought to have in common, as an important pain mechanism, *extra*cranial arterial vasodilation. The description of the vascular headaches of the migraine type as it appears in the NINDB classification is as follows: "Recurrent attacks of headache, widely varied in intensity, frequency, and duration. The attacks are commonly unilateral in onset; are usually associated with anorexia and, sometimes, with nausea and vomiting; in some are preceded by, or associated with, conspicuous sensory, motor, and mood disturbances; and are often familial."

In the headache classification as proposed by the International Headache Society (IHS) in 1988, migraine represents a separate category.[4] In this category, seven forms of migraine are distinguished as shown in Table 1.1. The two major forms of migraine in this classification, migraine without aura and migraine with aura, correspond with common and classic migraine of the NINDB classification.

TABLE 1.1
IHS classification of migraine

1.1 Migraine without aura
1.2 Migraine with aura
    1.2.1 Migraine with typical aura
    1.2.2 Migraine with prolonged aura
    1.2.3 Familial hemiplegic migraine
    1.2.4 Basilar migraine
    1.2.5 Migraine aura without headache
    1.2.6 Migraine with acute onset aura
1.3 Ophthalmoplegic migraine
1.4 Retinal migraine
1.5 Childhood periodic syndromes that may be precursors to or associated with migraine
    1.5.1 Benign paroxysmal vertigo of childhood
    1.5.2 Alternating hemiplegia of childhood
1.6 Complications of migraine
    1.6.1 Status migrainosus
    1.6.2 Migrainous infarction
1.7 Migrainous disorders not fulfilling the above criteria

From the Headache Classification Committee of the International Headache Society, 1988 with permission.[4]

4   *Management of Migraine*

Diagnostic Criteria

In its classification, the IHS has proposed strict criteria for the diagnosis of the headache conditions included. However, though strict criteria are important in research, they are *not* important in patient care. In patient care, the IHS criteria should be taken only as guidelines, and clinical judgment should be used. With regard to the diagnosis of migraine without aura, the IHS classification requires at least five attacks which fulfill the following criteria: (1) The headaches last from between 4 and 72 hours (though in children below the age of 15, they may last for as little as 2 hours). (2) The headaches have at least two of the following four features: unilateral location, pulsating quality, moderate or severe intensity, and aggravation by walking stairs or similar routine physical activity. The intensity of the headaches is rated as moderate when they *inhibit* and severe when they *prohibit* daily activities. (3) The headaches are associated with nausea or vomiting or with photo- *and* phonophobia (i.e., light and noise sensitivity).

The diagnosis of migraine with aura is based on the aura symptoms and *not* on the headache (i.e., the features of the headache are irrelevant (sic!). The IHS classification requires at least two attacks which fulfill three of the following four criteria: (1) There are one or more fully reversible aura symptoms, indicating focal cerebrocortical or brain-stem dysfunction. (2) At least one of the aura symptoms develops gradually over more than four minutes, or two or more symptoms occur in succession. (3) None of the aura symptoms last longer than 60 minutes but if more than one aura symptom is present, the accepted duration is proportionally increased. (4) The headache follows the aura symptoms with a symptom-free interval of less than 60 minutes but may also begin before or simultaneously with the aura.

In general practice, the various subgroups of migraine with aura are probably of little significance. An exception is the subgroup *migraine aura without headache* (1.2.5) in which the aura symptoms are *not* followed by headache. This is a relatively common condition which in the older patient needs to be differentiated from transient ischemic attacks.

In *migraine with prolonged aura* (1.2.2), one or more of the aura symptoms last longer than 60 minutes but shorter than one week, and neuroimaging is normal. If neuroimaging is abnormal (i.e., shows ischemic infarction) or one or more of the aura symptoms lasts longer than one week, *migrainous infarction* is diagnosed (1.6.2). Migrainous infarction is a subgroup of complications of migraine (1.6) and can occur in migraine without aura as well. It is also referred to as *complicated migraine* or *migraine complicated by stroke*.

In *migraine with acute onset aura* (1.2.6), the aura symptoms develop fully within four minutes. However, inaccurate history is given as the most common reason for the acute onset of the aura symptoms.

Familial hemiplegic migraine (1.2.3) is a rare (childhood) condition of headaches associated with hemiparesis, in which at least one first-degree relative is also affected.

Basilar migraine (1.2.4) is likewise a rare condition that mostly affects young adults. In this condition, the aura symptoms (e.g., double vision, bilateral paresthesias, or decreased level of arousal) originate from the brain stem or from *both* occipital lobes. The condition must be differentiated from migraine associated with anxiety and hyperventilation or with vasovagal lability.

Retinal migraine (1.4) is a form of migraine with aura, although it is classified as a separate condition. The aura symptoms are visual in nature but are monocular rather than homonymous. They also are fully reversible, last less than 60 minutes, and are followed by headache with a symptom-free interval of less than 60 minutes.

In *ophthalmoplegic migraine* (1.3), the headaches are associated with paresis of one or more of the cranial ocular nerves (i.e., the oculomotor, trochlear, or abducens nerves). In the majority of cases, the oculomotor nerve is involved and often only the parasympathetic nerve fibers, resulting in a dilated pupil that is unresponsive to light.

Status migrainosus, or *migraine status* (1.6.1), is one of the two complications of migraine, the other being migrainous infarction (1.6.2). Status migrainosus is the term used for migraine headaches lasting longer than 72 hours, although a headache-free interval of less than four hours between consecutive headaches may occur. As with migrainous infarction, status migrainosus can occur in migraine without aura as well as in migraine with aura.

References

1. Spierings ELH. Episodic and chronic jabs and jolts syndrome. Headache Q 1990; 1:299–302.
2. Spierings ELH. Episodic and chronic paroxysmal hemicrania. Clin J Pain 1992; 8:44–48.
3. Committee on Classification of Headache of the National Institute of Neurological Diseases and Blindness. Classification of headache. JAMA 1962; 179:717–718.
4. Headache Classification Committee of the International Headache Society. Classification and diagnostic criteria for headache disorders, cranial neuralgias and facial pain. Cephalalgia 1988; 8 (suppl. 7): 1–96.

CHAPTER 2

Symptomatology and Pathogenesis

Symptomatology

The symptoms of migraine are limited mostly to the migraine attack; between the attacks, usually patients are relatively symptom-free. The central symptom of the migraine attack is headache, though it is sometimes absent (as in migraine aura without headache). The headache of migraine is usually so intense as to be associated with at least some degree of disability. Typically it is limited to one side of the head, but this is certainly not always the case. When limited to one side, the headache alternates sides, though it may exhibit a preference for one side or the other. Within the head, the headache of migraine is often located in the temple and sometimes also in or behind the eye. Other preferential locations of the migraine headache are in the forehead and in the back of the head, often just behind the ear. The headache is either throbbing or sharp-steady in nature, especially in the temple. It is aggravated by such physical activity as going up a flight of stairs, which also may bring out its throbbing nature. The same is often true for activities such as bending over, coughing, sneezing, or straining. The headache is generally alleviated somewhat by lying down and by applying pressure or a cold pack to the temple, eye, or forehead.

The migraine headache almost always occurs associated with other symptoms. These symptoms generally occur *after* the onset of the headache and build up in intensity as the headache progresses. The associated symptoms of the migraine headache can be divided into two groups: autonomic and sensory. The autonomic symptoms consist of pallor of the face, coldness of the hands and feet, lack of appetite, nausea, vomiting, and diarrhea. They are probably caused by excessive activation of the sympathetic nervous system, secondary to the pain.

The sensory symptoms consist of increased sensitivity to light, noise, and smell (i.e., photo-, phono-, and odorphobia). The increased sensitivity sometimes reaches a degree at which exposure to light or noise actually in-

8   *Management of Migraine*

creases the intensity of the pain. Similarly, increased sensitivity to smell can reach an extent at which exposure to an odor, even when pleasant (e.g., perfume), aggravates the intensity of the nausea and causes vomiting.

The cause of the sensory symptoms is not known, but they are probably also secondary to the headache. They may be due to the increased arousal caused by the pain through stimulation of the reticular activating system. However, in the increased sensitivity to light (photophobia), a peripheral mechanism also may be involved—possibly the relaxation of the muscles of accommodation through activation of the rudimentary sympathetic innervation of these muscles. Such a peripheral mechanism also may explain the blurring of vision, especially of near vision, as is regularly observed during migraine headaches. This blurring of vision often is not recognized as an associated symptom of migraine and is sometimes taken for a migraine aura symptom.

In so-called classic migraine or migraine with aura, the migraine headache is preceded by transient focal neurological symptoms. These symptoms are generally referred to as aura symptoms and are almost always sensory in nature. They occur before the onset of the headache or during the initial phase of headache development. They are relatively short in duration and generally last from 10 to 30 minutes. The aura symptoms of migraine are most often visual in nature but also can be somatosensory. The typical presentation of the visual aura of migraine is the *scintillating scotoma*, also referred to as "fortification spectra" or "teichopsia" (Figure 2.1). It usually begins near the center of vision as a twinkling star that develops into a circle of bright, sometimes colorful, flickering zigzag lines. The inside of the circle subsequently opens up and develops into a semicircle or horseshoe, which further expands into the periphery of one visual field. On the inside of the semicircle or horseshoe, a band of dimness follows in the wake of the crescent of flickering zigzag lines. The visual disturbance ultimately fades away in the periphery of the visual field in which it developed.

The typical presentation of the somatosensory disturbance of migraine is the *digitolingual syndrome* (Figure 2.1). It consists of a feeling of numbness or tingling that starts in the fingers of one hand. Subsequently, the numbness gradually extends upward into the arm and, at a certain point, also involves the nose-mouth area on the same side. The progression of the numbness, like that of the scintillating scotoma, is slow and usually takes from 10 to 30 minutes. The digitolingual syndrome is *always* unilateral and must be differentiated from the bilateral paresthesias of hyperventilation syndrome. Sometimes the numbness is so intense that the involved extremity is perceived as being weak, but examination will disprove this. If real muscle weakness occurs with migraine, the condition is either *hemiplegic migraine* or *migrainous infarction*. Hemiplegic migraine is a rare, familial condition of childhood; migrainous infarction is a migraine attack complicated by stroke. However, if a stroke occurs during a migraine attack, it usually results in homonymous hemianopia rather than in hemiparesis. The

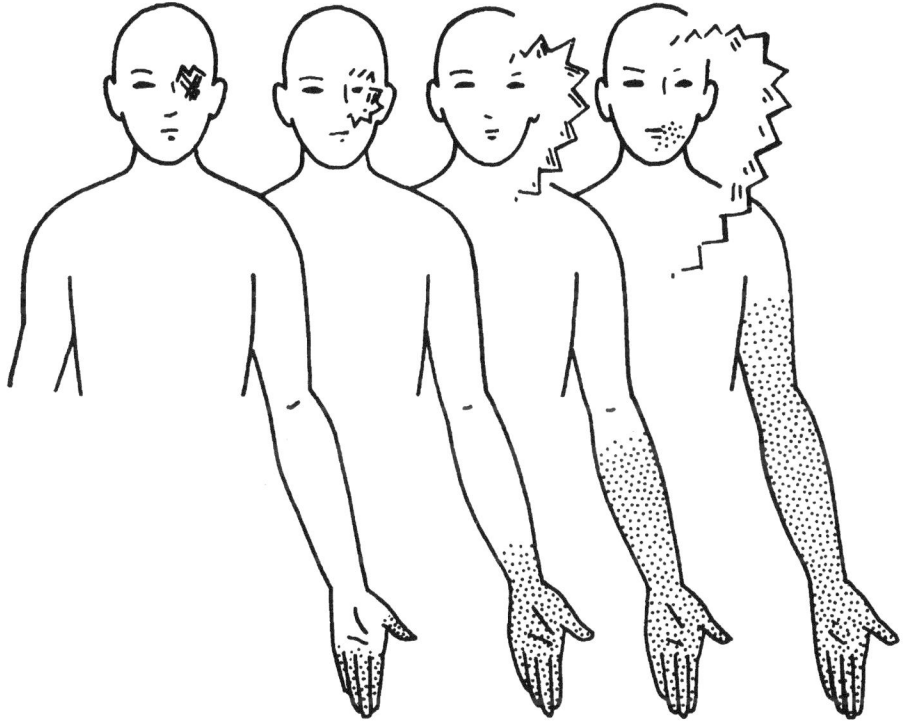

FIGURE 2.1 Scintillating scotoma (above) and digitolingual syndrome (below) from left to right in their successive stages of development.

occurrence of stroke with migraine is a one-time event and generally results in permanent symptoms.

Pathogenesis

Migraine headache

There is *clinical,* as opposed to animal, experimental, evidence that at least three mechanisms are involved in the pathogenesis of the migraine headache. These mechanisms are: *extra*cranial arterial vasodilation, *extra*cranial neurogenic inflammation, and decreased inhibition of central pain transmission.

The mechanism of *extracranial arterial vasodilation* was first studied in the 1930s by Graham and Wolff. They observed that pressure exerted on the extracranial arteries temporarily decreases the intensity of the pain.[1] In addition, they found that administration of ergotamine results in a decrease in intensity of the headaches, paralleling a decrease in pulsation amplitude

10   *Management of Migraine*

of the extracranial arteries. It was also observed that increasing the pressure of the cerebrospinal fluid by intrathecal injection of saline (thereby decreasing the pulsation amplitude of the cerebral arteries) does *not* decrease the intensity of the pain.[2]

The artery preferentially involved in the mechanism of extracranial arterial vasodilation is the frontal branch of the superficial temporal artery, giving rise to the pain in the temple, 50 characteristics of migraine. Regarding the involvement of this artery in the pathogenesis of the migraine headache, recent clinical experimental evidence showed that during the headache, the artery is relatively dilated on the side of the pain (Figure 2.2).[3] The dilation is relative, as there is generalized vasoconstriction during the migraine headache, probably caused by the increased activity of the sympathetic nervous system and responsible for the pallor of the face and coldness of the hands and feet.

Neurogenic inflammation is an inflammation caused by the release of chemicals from the primary sensory nerve fibers that are involved in pain

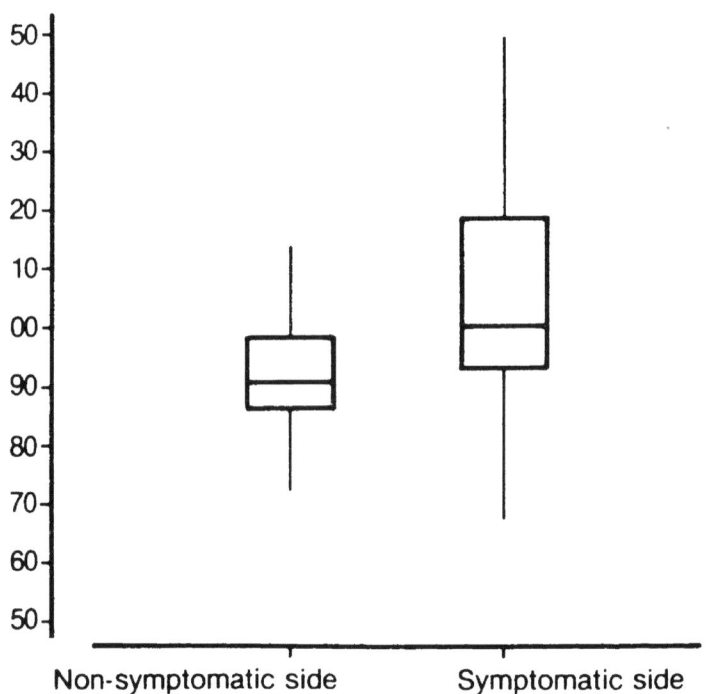

FIGURE 2.2   Luminal diameter of the frontal branch of the superficial temporal artery during attacks of migraine as a percentage of the diameter between attacks. From Iversen HK, Nielsen TH, Olesen J, Tfelt-Hansen P. Arterial responses during migraine headache. Lancet 1990; 336: 837–839 with permission.

transmission. These chemicals, which include substance P, calcitonin gene-related peptide, and neurokinin A, are released from the nerve fibers when they are activated. In migraine, the nerve fiber activation may be caused by the dilation of the extracranial arteries. Because the extracranial arteries have nerve fibers that coil around them, dilation results in stretching and, hence, activation of these nerve fibers. In the 1950s, Chapman and Wolff first studied neurogenic inflammation as a mechanism involved in the pathogenesis of the migraine headache. They observed that subcutaneous perfusates of the painful site have inflammatory activity proportional to the intensity of the pain (Figure 2.3).[4] In addition, they found that administration of ergotamine results in a decrease in inflammatory activity, parallel to a decrease in intensity of the pain. More recently, it has been observed that during the migraine headache, the level of calcitonin gene-related peptide is increased in the external jugular vein (Figure 2.4).[5] Calcitonin gene-related peptide is one of the chemicals involved in neurogenic inflammation, and the external jugular vein drains the *extra*cranial tissues.

Apart from neurogenic inflammation, there is probably also a *central mechanism* involved in the decrease in pain threshold at the site of the pain.

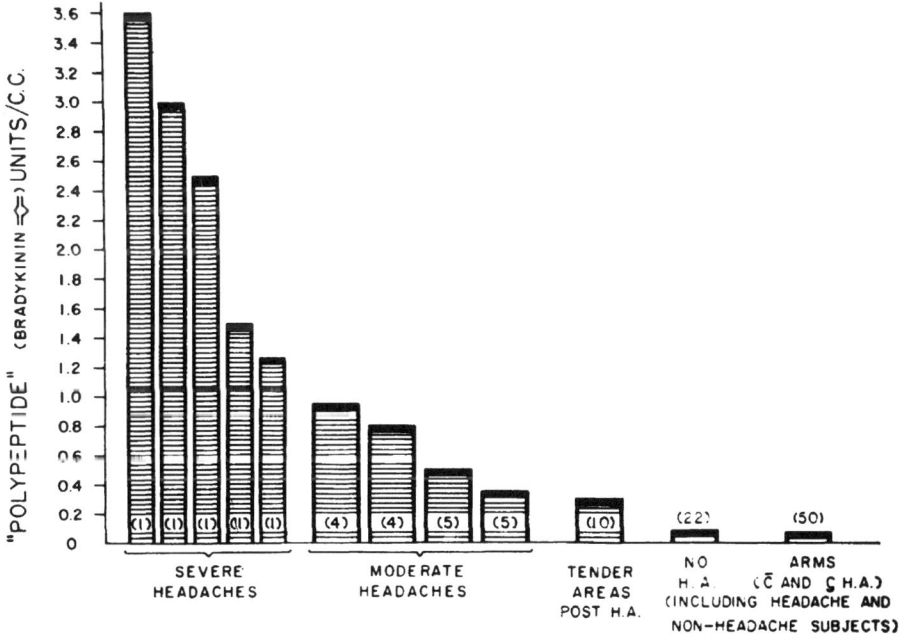

FIGURE 2.3 Inflammatory activity of subcutaneous perfusates of the site of the migraine headache, measured in bradykinin units, in relation to the intensity of the pain. From Chapman LF, et al. A humoral agent implicated in vascular headache of the migraine type. Arch Neurol 1960; 3:223–229 with permission.

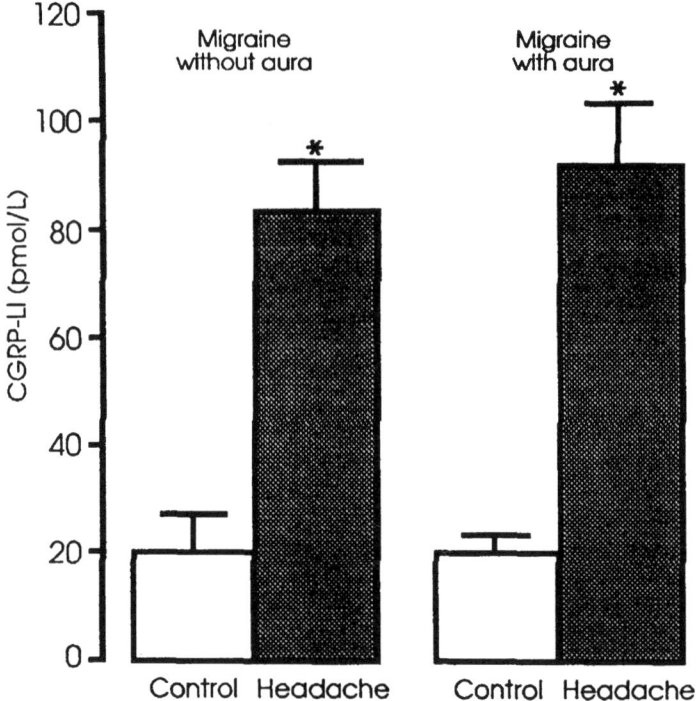

FIGURE 2.4 Levels of calcitonin gene-related peptide in blood drawn from the external jugular vein in controls and in patients with migraine with or without aura during the presence of headache. From Edvinsson L, Goadsby PJ. Neuropeptides in migraine and cluster headache. Cephalalgia 1994; 14: 320–327 with permission.

Evidence for this is provided by a study of the enkephalin level in the cerebrospinal fluid during the migraine headache. Enkephalin is an endogenous opioid which inhibits the transmission of pain signals in the central nervous system. Its level was found to be decreased during the migraine headache in comparison to the headache-free interval and in comparison to controls (Figure 2.5).[6]

Migraine aura

The pathogenesis of the migraine aura was first studied by Schumacher, Marcussen, and Wolff in the 1940s and 1950s. They observed that inhalation of a cerebral vasodilator (e.g., amyl nitrite or carbon dioxide) during the migraine aura results in a transient regression of the symptoms (Figure 2.6).[2,7] Hence, they concluded that the migraine aura is caused by transient cerebral vasoconstriction. In 1958, Milner reported on the similarities in features and

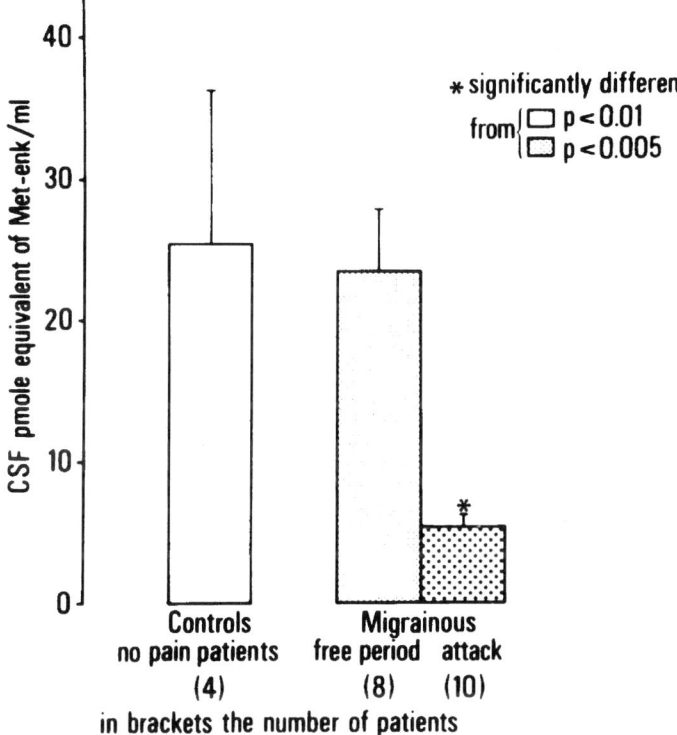

FIGURE 2.5 Enkephalin levels of the cerebrospinal fluid during and between migraine attacks and in control subjects. From Anselmi B, Baldi E, Casacci F, Salmon S. Endogenous opioids in cerebrospinal fluid and blood in idiopathic headache sufferers. Headache 1980; 20: 294–299 with permission.

progression between the scintillating scotoma and spreading depression, a neurophysiological phenomenon described by Leao in 1944.[8] Spreading depression is a wave of inhibition of the cortical neuronal activity, which travels over the cerebral cortex at a slow rate and is preceded by a short phase of intense neuronal activity.

In the 1970s, relatively accurate measurement of the cerebral blood flow became possible with the development of the Xenon clearance technique. Olesen et al. recently summarized the results of cerebral blood flow studies in 63 patients with classic migraine or migraine with aura.[9] It was concluded that the aura symptoms occur *after* cerebral blood flow decreases in the posterior region of the opposite hemisphere. The headache occurs while blood flow is still decreased but is associated with a gradual *increase* in cerebral blood flow to an abnormally high level (Figure 2.7). The increase in cerebral blood flow following the initial decrease probably reflects reac-

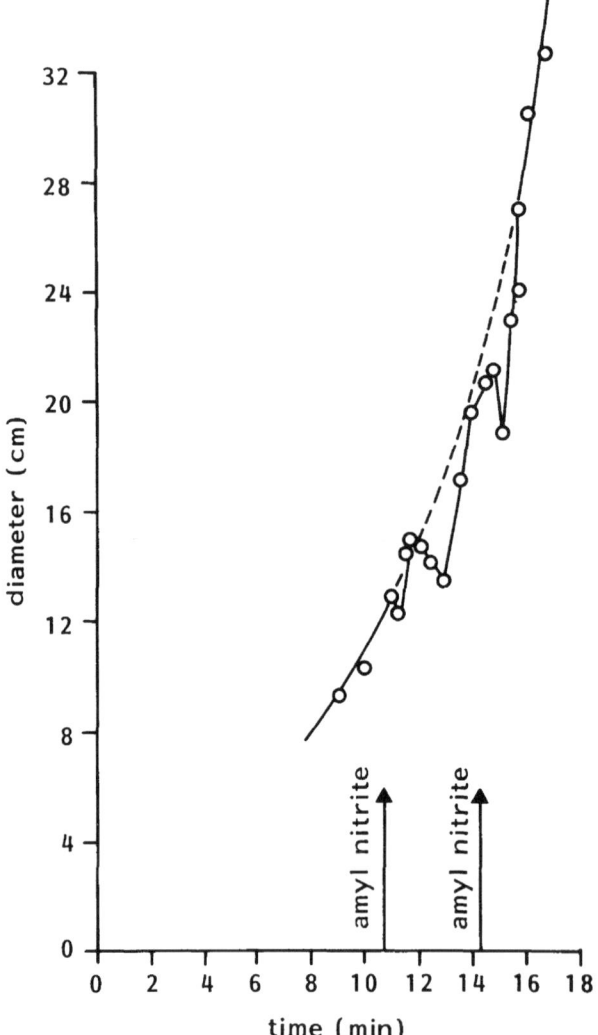

FIGURE 2.6 Effect of the cerebral vasodilator amyl nitrite on the progression of the scintillating scotoma. From Hare EH. Personal observations on the spectral march of migraine. J Neurol Sci 1966; 3: 259–264 with permission.

tive hyperemia, though it is not certain that the decrease in cerebral blood flow actually reaches ischemic levels. Initially, the decrease in cerebral blood flow of the migraine aura was described as an *oligemia,* which spread over the cerebral cortex at a slow rate similar to Leão's spreading depression (Figure 2.8).[10]

On the basis of the clinical presentation of the migraine aura, my choice of the mechanism involved is a phenomenon such as spreading depression rather than transient cerebral vasoconstriction. This notion is supported by the results of brain spectroscopy, which show an alteration in energy metabolism in patients with classic migraine or migraine with aura

Symptomatology and Pathogenesis 15

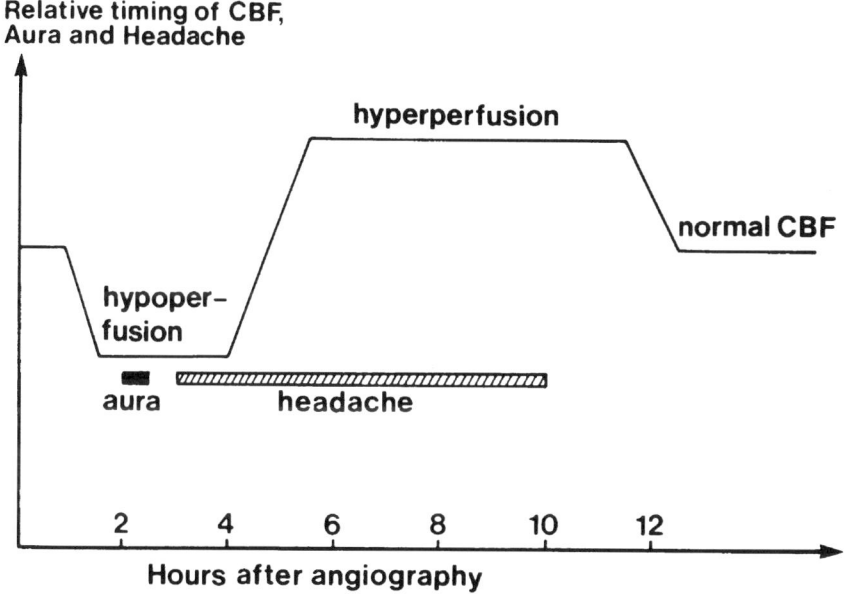

FIGURE 2.7 Changes in cerebral blood flow in relation to the occurrence of the aura and headache in attacks of migraine with aura. From Olesen J, Friberg L, Olsen TS, et al. Timing and topography of cerebral blood flow, aura, and headache during migraine attacks. Ann Neurol 1990; 28: 791–798 with permission.

but without changes in pH.[11] Cerebral vasoconstriction, in my opinion, is the mechanism involved in migrainous infarction or migraine complicated by stroke, which occurs in migraine *unrelated* to the occurrence of aura symptoms.[12]

Migraine attack

It must be remembered that only in a minority of cases is the migraine headache preceded by an aura. In the majority (i.e., in common migraine or migraine without aura), the migraine headache occurs without an aura but is, nevertheless, otherwise the same. In the traditional view, the pathogenesis of the migraine aura and headache are causally related, that is, the aura is considered to be the cause of the headache. The aura is related to cerebral vasoconstriction, which causes hypoxia of the brain and is followed by reactive vasodilation. The vasodilation occurs in the cerebral circulation but is associated with a dilation of *extra*cranial arteries. The extracranial arterial vasodilation initiates the neurogenic inflammation, and the combination of the two mechanisms causes the migraine headache (Figure 2.9).

16   *Management of Migraine*

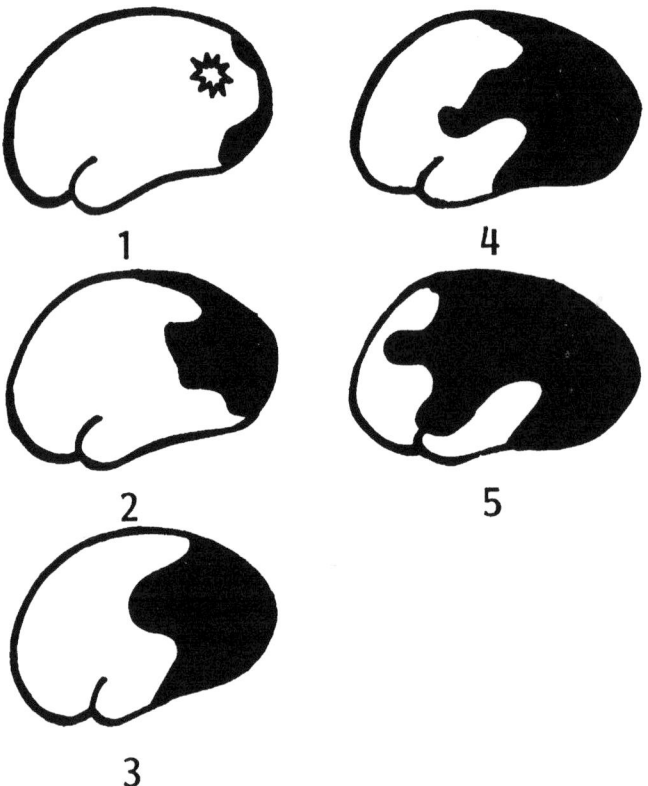

FIGURE 2.8   Changes in cerebral blood flow of the migraine aura described as spreading oligemia. Adapted from Olesen J, Larsen B, Lauritzen M. Focal hyperemia followed by spreading oligemia and impaired activation of rCBF in classic migraine. Ann Neurol 1981; 9: 344–352 with permission.

In common migraine or migraine without aura, the cerebral vasoconstriction and hypoxia are thought to occur as well but in a clinically silent area of the cerebral cortex. However, there is no evidence for this assumption, nor is there evidence that cerebral vasodilation is associated with a dilation of extracranial arteries. The two assumptions were made to connect the migraine aura with the headache in a causal way and to bring the two forms of migraine (i.e., migraine with and without aura) together in one pathogenetic concept. However, the migraine aura and headache may *not* be causally related, and the two forms of migraine may *not* share the same pathogenesis. On the basis of the results of the cerebral blood flow studies, at least it can be stated that the aura and headache are *not* causally related through cerebral vasodilation, as the cerebral vasodilation occurs *after* the onset of the headache.

Symptomatology and Pathogenesis   17

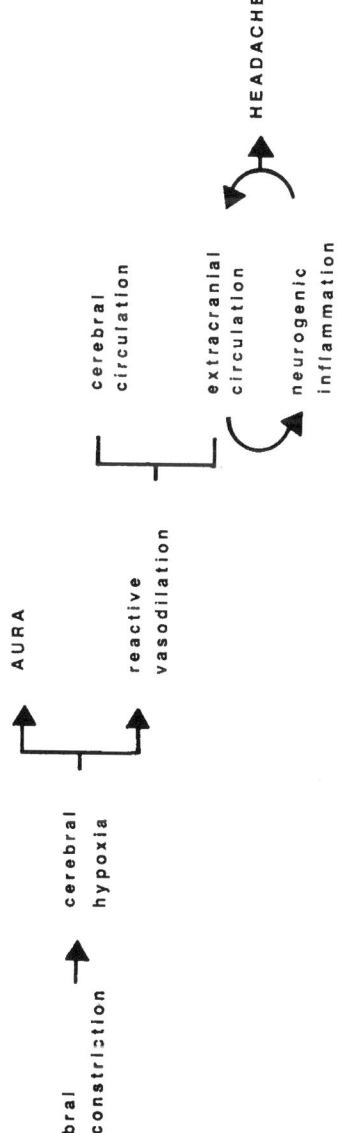

FIGURE 2.9   Traditional view on the pathogenesis of the migraine attack in which the aura and headache are considered sequential phenomena.

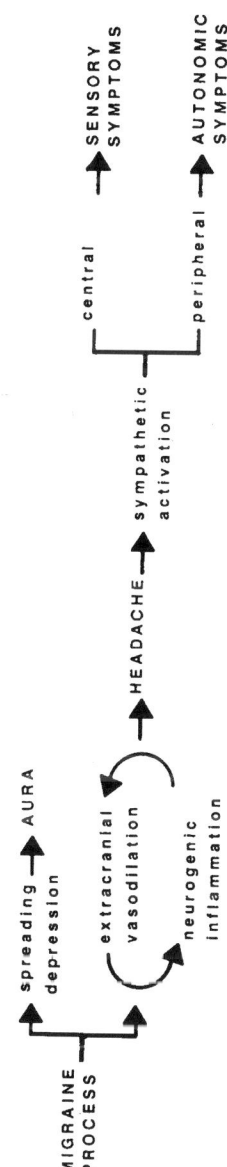

FIGURE 2.10   Alternative view on the pathogenesis of the migraine attack in which the aura and headache are considered parallel phenomena, and the associated symptoms of the migraine headache secondary to the pain.

Except for the aura, the clinical presentations of migraine with and without aura are so similar that a common pathogenesis is plausible. Also, the two forms of migraine very often occur in the same individual, with headaches preceded by an aura at some times but not at other times. Although the aura often occurs before the onset of the headache, this does not mean , therefore, that the aura is necessarily the *cause* of the headache. The particular time relationship between the occurrence of the aura and headache also can be explained in other ways. For example, it can be explained by the greater reactivity of the cerebral tissues, as compared to the extracranial tissues, in giving rise to symptoms when the physiology is disturbed.

In the alternative concept, the pathogenesis of the migraine aura and headache are considered parallel rather than sequential in nature (Figure 2.10). They are joined by what I have referred to as the *migraine process*, the driving force behind the migraine attack which is activated by the migraine trigger factors. The concept better explains the isolated occurrence of the migraine aura (i.e., migraine aura without headache) and the isolated occurrence of the migraine headache (i.e., migraine without aura). The concept also includes the associated symptoms of the migraine headache (i.e., the autonomic and sensory symptoms) as secondary to the headache through stimulation of the sympathetic nervous system and reticular activating system, respectively.

References

1. Graham JR, Wolff HG. Mechanism of migraine headache and action of ergotamine tartrate. Arch Neurol Psychiatry 1938; 39:737–763.
2. Schumacher GA, Wolff HG . Experimental studies on headache. A. Contrast of histamine headache with the headache of migraine and that associated with hypertension. B. Contrast of vascular mechanisms in preheadache and in headache phenomena of migraine. Arch Neurol Psychiatry 1941; 45:199–214.
3. Iversen HK, Nielsen TH, Olesen J, Tfelt-Hansen P. Arterial responses during migraine headache. Lancet 1990; 336:837–839.
4. Chapman LF, Ramos AO, Goodell H, et al. A humoral agent implicated in vascular headache of the migraine type. Arch Neurol 1960; 3:223–229.
5. Goadsby PJ, Edvinsson L, Ekman R. Vasoactive peptide release in the extracerebral circulation of humans during migraine headache. Ann Neurol 1990; 28:183–187.
6. Anselmi B, Baldi E, Casacci F, Salmon S. Endogenous opioids in cerebrospinal fluid and blood in idiopathic headache sufferers. Headache 1980; 20:294–299.
7. Marcussen RM, Wolff HG. Studies on headache. 1. Effects of carbon dioxide-oxygen mixtures given during preheadache phase of the migraine attack. 2. Further analysis of the pain mechanisms in headache. Arch Neurol Psychiatry 1950; 63:42–51.
8. Milner PM. Note on a possible correspondence between the scotomas of migraine and spreading depression of Leão. Electroencephalogr Clin Neurophysiol 1958; 10:705.

9. Olesen J, Friberg L, Olsen TS, et al. Timing and topography of cerebral blood flow, aura, and headache during migraine attacks. Ann Neurol 1990; 28:791–798.
10. Olesen J, Larsen B, Lauritzen M. Focal hyperemia followed by spreading oligemia and impaired activation of rCBF in classic migraine. Ann Neurol 1981; 9: 344–352.
11. Welch KMA, Levine SR, D'Andrea G, et al. Preliminary observations on brain energy metabolism in migraine studied by in vivo phosphorus 31 NMR spectroscopy. Neurology 1989; 39:538–541.
12. Spierings ELH. Angiographic changes suggestive of vasospasm in migraine complicated by stroke. Headache 1990; 30:727–728.

CHAPTER 3

Diagnosis and Differential Diagnosis

Diagnosis

Migraine is a chronic condition of recurring headaches; therefore, the diagnosis should be considered in cases of recurring headaches. Sometimes migraine manifests itself only in recurring transient focal neurological symptoms (i.e., isolated migraine aura or migraine aura without headache). For that reason, the diagnosis of migraine should also be considered in cases of recurring neurological symptoms. However, the neurological symptoms would have to be sensory in nature, either visual or somatosensory, and fully reversible. They typically develop slowly (i.e., over minutes) and last from 10 to 30 minutes. They are often presented as loss of function (i.e., loss of vision or loss of sensation) though actually the function is *not* lost but disturbed. Hence, the symptoms are those of disturbed vision (i.e., scintillations in one or both visual fields) or disturbed somatosensation (i.e., paresthesias in one or the other side of the body).

Similar sensory symptoms are seen with focal (occipital- or temporal-lobe) epilepsy. However, in epilepsy, the symptoms progress over seconds and are followed by loss of consciousness due to generalization of the seizure activity. The transient focal neurological symptoms encountered in transient ischemic attacks differ in other ways. They truly represent loss of function, come about suddenly without progression, and last for seconds or minutes.

The diagnosis of migraine in acute, severe headache should be considered only when there is a prior history of similar headaches. In the presence of fever, meningitis (either viral or bacterial) is an important diagnosis to contemplate. Meningitis occurs mostly before the age of 20 and is a particularly significant consideration in children with acute, severe headache. The patient with bacterial meningitis is generally very sick and may be delirious. However, a case of viral meningitis can be easily mistaken for migraine.

Acute, severe headache without fever creates suspicion for intracranial hemorrhage, especially subarachnoid hemorrhage. The headache caused by intracranial hemorrhage occurs in a very sudden onset, coming about in a matter of seconds. Therefore, in a patient with acute, severe headache, the onset of headache should always be established as precisely as possible. The headache of migraine comes about relatively slowly, requiring one or more hours to build up to its maximum intensity. The headache of cluster headache builds up to its maximum intensity more rapidly but still requires minutes.

In a *prospective* study, 27 patients who presented acute severe headache were subjected to computerized tomography, if negative, followed by lumbar puncture.[1] The patients did not exhibit an obvious cause of the headaches, did *not* have prior history of similar headaches, and did *not* show focal neurological symptoms or signs. Subarachnoid hermorrhage was diagnosed in nine of the patients (in four through computerized tomography and in five through lumbar puncture) and menigitis in two.

The most noticeable diagnostic feature of migraine is recurring headaches of moderate or severe intensity. Between the headaches, the patient is relatively symptom-free, and this should be ascertained in the history. If headaches do occur frequently between the migraine headaches, the diagnosis of chronic daily headache should be considered (*vide infra*).

The frequency of migraine headache occurrence varies greatly, from once per year to once or twice per week. However, when the headaches occur frequently (i.e., once per week or more), the diagnosis of chronic daily headache should again be considered. Also, the duration of migraine headaches varies greatly, but minimally they last from four to six hours, although in children they can be shorter. According to the diagnostic criteria of the International Headache Society (IHS), the maximum duration of the migraine headache is 72 hours, after which it is referred to as *status migrainosus* (*migraine status*). However, migraine headaches can continue for days and still terminate by themselves, a phenomenon seen particularly in menstrual migraine.

Migraine headaches come about during the day or are present on awakening in the morning. They sometimes wake the patient at night, and if this occurs, it happens in the early morning hours (i.e., between 4 and 6 AM). If the headaches occur regularly (i.e., on a weekly basis) and wake the patient in the early morning, chronic daily headache again should be considered. Only the headaches of cluster headache wake the patient in the early hours of the night (i.e., between midnight and 2 AM). Migraine headaches can be present in their full intensity on awakening in the morning or when they wake the patient at night; otherwise, they generally require at least several hours to build up to their maximum intensity.

About two-thirds of migraine headaches are limited to one side of the head. Typically, the headaches alternate between the two sides of the head, though they often have a preference for one side or the other. When the headaches *always* occur on the same side (i.e., always on the right or always on the left), an explanation is required. The explanation can be a structural, intracranial lesion, as in so-called symptomatic migraine (vide infra). However, the explanation also can be another type of asymmetric abnormality of the head, face, or neck. Such an asymmetric abnormality can be a chronic ipsilateral maxillary sinusitis or chronic spasm of the ipsilateral posterior cervical muscles.

Within the head, the migraine headache is often localized, generally to the temple, eye, or forehead but sometimes to the back of the head. It is typically dull-throbbing or sharp-steady in nature and becomes worse with physical activity, moving around, bending over, straining, coughing, and so on. Lying down quietly, preferably in a dark and quiet room, sometimes with the head slightly elevated, often alleviates the headache somewhat. Also, applying pressure on the temple(s) or a cold cloth over the forehead often provides some temporary relief of the pain. The migraine headache is almost always associated with other symptoms, the gastrointestinal symptoms being generally most prominent, ranging from lack of appetite to vomiting. There is generally also increased sensitivity of the sensory organs, progressing from photophobia to phonophobia to odorphobia. The photo- and phonophobia can be so intense that exposure to light or noise aggravate the intensity of the pain. The odorphobia is often connected with the gastrointestinal symptoms, and they are, consequently, made worse by exposure to smells.

Chronic Daily Headache

Chronic daily headache is a descriptive term for the daily or almost daily occurrence of headaches. The high frequency of occurrence of the headaches is often not evident until the specific question is raised, especially in patients with severe headaches. This question must be raised in patients who have experienced the onset of migraine later in life (after the age of 30) or who have the headaches frequently (i.e., once per week or more).

Within chronic daily headache, two conditions can be distinguished: *tension-type vascular headache* and *chronic tension-type headache.* Tension-type vascular headache is not included in the classification of the IHS, as it is thought to be a combination of two conditions—chronic tension-type headache and migraine. Tension-type headache is the term used in the classification for muscle-contraction headache. However, most patients with tension-type vascular headache do not have two but one condition, and its origin may be either migraine or tension-type headache.

The interrelation of migraine, tension-type (muscle-contraction) vascular headache and tension-type (muscle-contraction) headache is shown in Figure 3.1. In the figure, tension-type headache is again divided into two conditions: *episodic* and *chronic* tension-type headache, depending on the

24 *Management of Migraine*

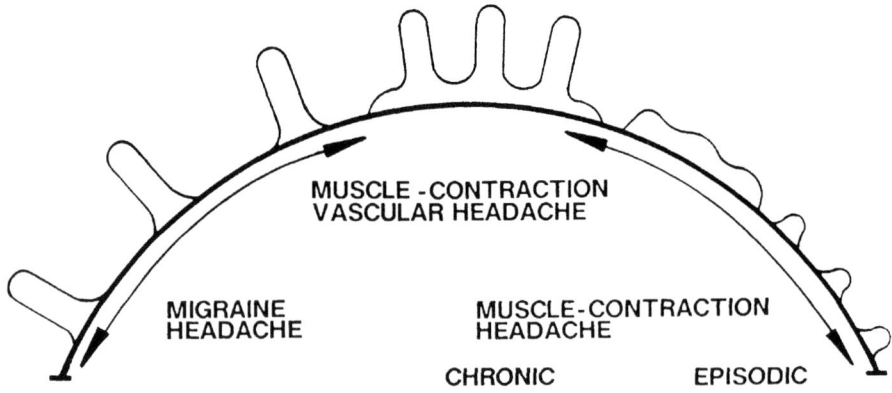

FIGURE 3.1 Interrelation of the major headache syndromes: episodic and chronic muscle-contraction (tension-type) headache, muscle-contraction (tension-type) vascular headache, and migraine.

frequency of occurrence of the headaches. In episodic tension-type headache, the headaches occur intermittently up to two or three times per week, whereas in chronic tension-type headache, they occur daily or almost daily. As opposed to migraine, the headaches of tension-type headache are mild to moderate in intensity and, therefore, generally *not* associated with other symptoms. Consequently, it is usually not difficult to distinguish migraine from tension-type headache.

This is different with migraine and tension-type vascular headache, because in both conditions the occurring migraine headaches are indistinguishable from each other. As the figure illustrates, the difference is that in migraine the patient is more or less symptom-free between the headaches, whereas in tension-type vascular headache, the patient has headaches all the time or almost all the time. It is necessary to distinguish between migraine and tension-type vascular headache, as a subgroup of patients with tension-type vascular headache do *not* have migraine. The headache condition in these patients developed out of tension-type headache (as the arrow on the right side of Figure 3.1 indicates).

Symptomatic Migraine

Symptomatic migraine is a condition which manifests itself as migraine but is caused by a structural, intracranial lesion. As migraine is a chronic condition, the intracranial lesions that cause symptomatic migraine are either not progressive or slowly progressive. Arteriovenous malformations and meningiomas are examples of lesions that can manifest themselves as migraine.

A feature to look for as an indication of symptomatic migraine is fixed and crossed lateralization of the headaches and the neurological symptoms. This means that the headaches *always* occur on the same side of the head and the neurological symptoms *always* on the opposite side. Another feature to look for is the persistence of neurological symptoms or signs between the headaches.

Complicated Migraine

Complicated migraine is a migraine attack which is complicated by ischemic stroke. According to the IHS classification, this complication occurs only in classic migraine or migraine with aura. However, this is not correct; the occurrence of stroke in migraine is independent of the occurrence of aura symptoms. It is more clearly related to the intensity of the headache and of its associated symptoms, nausea and vomiting. The pathogenesis of the ischemic stroke is likely also different from that of the aura symptoms. The migraine aura is probably caused by a primary neuronal disturbance, whereas the ischemic stroke is caused by cerebral vasospasm.[2]

References

1. Llede A, Calandre L, Martinez-Menedez B, et al. Acute headache of recent onset and subarachnoid hemorrage: A prospective study. Headache 1994; 34:172–174.
2. Spierings ELH. Angiographic changes suggestive of vasospasm in migraine complicated by stroke. Headache 1990; 30:727–728.

CHAPTER 4

Abortive Pharmacological Treatment

Abortive treatment refers to treatment of the individual migraine attack. It generally addresses the headache and aims at decreasing its intensity, if possible, to the extent that it is eliminated fully. With effective reduction in headache intensity, there is generally also a decrease in intensity of such associated symptoms as nausea, vomiting, photo- and phonophobia, as they occur secondary to the pain. The gastrointestinal symptoms also can be addressed directly with antinausea medications. There are no specific treatments for the sensory symptoms (i.e., photo- and phonophobia), but they may be relieved by accommodating the patient in a dark and quiet room. Lying down, sometimes with the head elevated, often also decreases the intensity of the headache and may help to reduce the nausea and vomiting as well. Cold applied to the head, especially to the forehead and temple(s), and sometimes pressure applied to the temple(s) are additional measures to decrease the intensity of the pain.

With regard to the migraine aura, inhalation of carbon dioxide and rebreathing of air were studied in small, *open* trials and found to be modestly effective.[1] Domperidone (Motilium, UK; not available in the US) is the only treatment of the migraine aura which was studied in a double-blind, placebo-controlled trial.[2] The trial used a *crossover* design and involved 19 patients. The dose of the medication was 30 mg by mouth, taken at the onset of the aura. The medication was effective in relieving the aura and preventing the headache in 66 percent of the attacks treated. On the other hand, treatment with placebo relieved the aura and prevented the headache in only 5 percent. I have observed similar effects of metoclopramide (Maxolon or Primperan, UK; Reglan, US) which, like domperidone, is a dopamine-2-receptor antagonist and a gastrokinetic antiemetic.

Generally, abortive treatment always is indicated, as the migraine headache is usually so intense that it interferes with the ability to function. However, not only the intensity of the headache causes the disability, but the associated gastrointestinal symptoms contribute as well. Actually, it is often the occurrence of nausea that forces the patient to lie down, as motion tends to aggravate the gastrointestinal symptoms. There are many antiemetic medications available to treat the gastrointestinal symptoms of migraine and they should be used whenever possible (Table 4.1).

The above mentioned medications, domperidone and metoclopramide, are so-called gastrokinetic antiemetics. They not only treat nausea and vomiting but also stimulate the activity of the gastrointestinal tract. The latter feature is important in migraine, as the headache is associated with abnormal functioning of the gastrointestinal tract, which impairs the absorption of oral medications (*vide infra*). An additional advantage of the medications is that they generally do not cause drowsiness, which is important as they have to be taken early in the onset of the attack.

The usual dose of either medication is 10 or 20 mg by mouth, as needed for nausea every four to six hours. Metoclopramide, as opposed to domperidone, passes the blood-brain barrier and, therefore, can cause akathesia and, rarely, dystonia. These adverse effects occur particularly in adolescents and young adults and are more common in women than in men. The akathesia consists of restlessness and the dystonia often affects the tongue, which feels swollen and stiff. The symptoms can be reversed by administration of an anticholinergic medication such as diphenhydramine (Benadryl, UK/US), 25 or 50 mg intravenously.

For the abortive treatment of the migraine headache, two types of medications can be used: *analgesics* and *vasoconstrictors*. As the vasoconstrictors are more specific for migraine, they are generally also more effective.

The analgesics are traditionally divided into three groups: *simple analgesics*, *nonsteroidal anti-inflammatory analgesics* and *narcotic analgesics*. Migraine is a chronic, often lifelong condition; therefore, the use of such po-

TABLE 4.1
Medications for the treatment of nausea and vomiting

Anticholinergic antiemetics
   Trimethobenzamide (Tigan, UK/US)
Antidopaminergic antiemetics
   Chlorpromazine (Thorazine, UK/US)
   Prochlorperazine (Stemetil, UK; Compazine, US)
   Thiethylperazine (not available in the UK; Torecan, US)
Antihistaminergic antiemetics
   Diphenhydramine (Benadryl, UK/US)
   Hydroxyzine (Atarax, UK; Vistaril, US)
   Promethazine (Phenergan, UK/US)
Gastrokinetic antiemetics
   Domperidone (Motilium, UK; not available in the US)
   Metoclopramide (Maxolon or Primperan, UK; Reglan, US)

tentially addicting medications as narcotic analgesics should be avoided. Also, in general, more effective relief of the migraine headache can be obtained with specific medications (i.e., with vasoconstrictors). The vasoconstrictor used most commonly for the abortive treatment of migraine is *caffeine*, either alone, such as in a strong cup of coffee (a home remedy for migraine) or in combination with other medications. With regard to the combination preparations containing caffeine, the medication has been shown to increase the analgesic potency of these preparations by 40 percent.[3]

Simple Analgesics

The so-called simple analgesics are aspirin (acetylsalicylic acid), acetaminophen (paracetamol), and ibuprofen. A summary of their reported efficacies in the abortive treatment of migraine is presented in Table 4.2.

TABLE 4.2
Reported efficacies of the simple analgesics in the abortive treatment of migraine

Analgesic	Efficacy	Study
Aspirin		
650 mg	42 percent improved or relieved	Tfelt-Hansen & Olesen, 1984[4]
1,000 mg	52 percent (almost) completely relieved	Boureau et al., 1994[5]
900 mg with 10 mg metoclopramide	34–45 percent efficacy* within 2 hours	Oral Sumatriptan and Aspirin plus Metoclopramide Comparative Study Group, 1992[59]
900 mg with 10 mg metoclopramide	56 percent efficacy* within two hours	Chabriat et al., 1994[7]
Ibuprofen		
800–1,200 mg	Duration 56 percent shorter than with placebo treatment	Havanka-Kanniainen, 1989[8]
1,200 mg	Intensity 24 percent lower and duration 34 percent shorter than with placebo treatment	Kloster et al., 1992[9]

*Defined as a reduction in headache intensity from moderate or severe to mild or no headache.

Aspirin

Aspirin was studied in two double-blind, placebo-controlled, *crossover* trials. The first trial involved 118 patients, 85 of whom completed the study.[4] The dose of the medication was 650 mg in an effervescent tablet that was taken at the onset of the headache. The medication improved 24 percent of the migraine headaches and relieved 18 percent (i.e., the total response rate was 42 percent). Treatment with placebo improved 15 percent of the headaches and relieved 5 percent (i.e., the total response rate was 20 percent).

The second trial involved 259 patients, 198 of whom completed the study.[5] The dose of the medication was 1,000 mg by mouth. Two hours after treatment, 52 percent of the patients obtained almost complete or complete relief of the headache as compared to 30 percent with placebo.

Aspirin was compared with *acetaminophen* in a double-blind, placebo-controlled, *parallel* study.[6] The trial involved 162 patients with tension-type vascular headache. The dose of aspirin was 650 mg by mouth and of acetaminophen, 1,000 mg. Aspirin was significantly better than placebo *two* hours after treatment, whereas acetaminophen was not. However, a direct comparison between the two medications did *not* show a statistically significant difference.

The combination of aspirin with metoclopramide was studied in a double-blind, placebo-controlled, *parallel* trial.[7] The trial involved 266 patients, 250 of whom completed the study. The dose of the aspirin was 900 mg (in the form of the highly soluble aspirin salt, lysine acetylsalicylate) and that of metoclopramide 10 mg. Efficacy was defined as a reduction in headache intensity from moderate or severe to mild or no headache. After two hours of treatment, efficacy was achieved in 56 percent of the headaches treated with the aspirin/metoclopramide combination and in 28 percent of those treated with placebo. Adverse effects were minor and transient and consisted of constipation, fatigue, lightheadedness, and vertigo.

Ibuprofen

Ibuprofen was studied in two double-blind, placebo-controlled, *crossover* trials. The first trial involved 40 patients, 27 of whom completed the study.[8] The dose of the medication was 800 mg by mouth, followed if necessary by another 400 mg after one-half to one hour. The duration of the headaches when treated with ibuprofen was 56 percent shorter than with placebo treatment and the incidence of severe headaches was 46 percent lower.

The second trial involved 36 patients, 25 of whom completed the study.[9] The dose of the medication was 1,200 mg by mouth. When treated with ibuprofen, the intensity of the headaches was 24 percent lower than with placebo treatment and their duration was 34 percent shorter.

Ibuprofen was compared with acetaminophen in a double-blind, *crossover* study.[10] The trial involved 30 patients, 22 of whom completed the study. The medications were provided in capsules containing 200 mg ibuprofen or 450 mg acetaminophen. The patients took two capsules at the onset of the headache, followed if necessary by two capsules as needed every four to six hours with a maximum of eight. Both medications decreased the intensity of the headaches, but ibuprofen also decreased their duration.

The efficacy of the simple analgesics often can be increased by combining them with a gastrokinetic medication (e.g., domperidone or metoclopramide). As mentioned earlier, these medications not only relieve nausea and vomiting but also stimulate the activity of the gastrointestinal tract, thereby improving the absorption of oral medications.

Domperidone

Domperidone was studied in a double-blind, placebo-controlled, *crossover* trial.[11] The trial involved 59 patients, 46 of whom completed the study. The dose of the medication was 20 or 30 mg by mouth, taken together with 1,000 mg acetaminophen. Domperidone increased the efficacy of the acetaminophen in decreasing the duration of the headaches by 31 percent but did not affect the effect of acetaminophem or the intensity of the headaches.

Metoclopramide

Metoclopramide was studied in a double-blind, placebo-controlled, *parallel* trial.[12] The trial involved 150 patients, 136 of whom completed the study. The dose of the medication was 20 mg by rectum, taken together with 1,000 mg acetaminophen and 5 mg diazepam by mouth (Valium, UK/US). Metoclopramide combined with acetaminophen and diazepam increased the excellent response of the headaches to the latter two medications from 38 to 59 percent.

Nonsteroidal Anti-Inflammatory Analgesics

Of the nonsteroidal anti-inflammatory analgesics, diclofenac, indomethacin, naproxen sodium, and tolfenamic acid were studied in the abortive treatment of migraine (Table 4.3). A summary of their reported efficacies is presented in Table 4.4.

Diclofenac

Diclofenac (Voltarol, UK; Voltaren, US) was studied in two double-blind, placebo-controlled, *crossover* trials. The first trial involved 107 patients, 104 of whom completed the study.[13] The dose of the medication was 50 mg by

TABLE 4.3
Nonsteroidal anti-inflammatory analgesics studied in the abortive treatment of migraine

Acetic acids
   Diclofenac (Voltarol, UK; Voltaren, US)
   Indomethacin (Indocid, UK; Indocin, US)
Propionic acids
   Naproxen sodium (Synflex, UK; Anaprox, US)
Anthranilic acids
   Tolfenamic acid (not available in the UK or US)

TABLE 4.4
Reported efficacies of the nonsteroidal anti-inflammatory analgesics in the abortive treatment of migraine

Analgesic	Efficacy	Study
Diclofenac		
50–100 mg	27 percent aborted within 2 hours	Massiou et al., 1991[13]
50 mg	39 percent efficacy* within 2 hours	Dahlof & Bjorkman, 1993[14]
100 mg	44 percent efficacy* within 2 hours	Dahlof & Bjorkman, 1993[14]
Naproxen Sodium		
825–1,375 mg	Intensity 24 percent lower and duration 20 percent shorter than with placebo treatment	Johnson et al., 1985[18]
750–1,750 mg	54 percent good or better than good response	Treves et al., 1992[19]
825–1,375 mg	31 percent decrease in headache intensity	Pradalier et al., 1985[21]
Tolfenamic acid		
200 mg	Duration 55 percent shorter than with placebo treatment	Hakkarainen et al., 1979[23]
200–400 mg	Duration 37 percent shorter than with placebo treatment	Tokola et al., 1984[72]

*Defined as a reduction in headache intensity from moderate or severe to mild or no headache.

mouth, taken within a half hour of the onset of the headache and repeated if necessary after one hour. Twenty-seven percent of the attacks were aborted within two hours when treated with diclofenac and 19 percent had the same results with placebo treatment. The intensity of the headaches was decreased by 12 percent when they were treated with the medication, whereas placebo treatment reduced the intensity by 5 percent.

The second trial involved 72 patients, 64 of whom completed the study.[14] The patients took the medication in a dose of 50 or 100 mg by mouth at the onset of the headache. The efficacy of diclofenac was 39 percent in the dose of 50 mg and 44 percent in the dose of 100 mg, whereas the placebo response was 22 percent (Figure 4.1). Efficacy was defined as a reduction in headache intensity from moderate or severe to mild or no headache within *two* hours of treatment. Adverse effects were experienced by 20 percent of the patients and were equally common with the medication as with placebo.

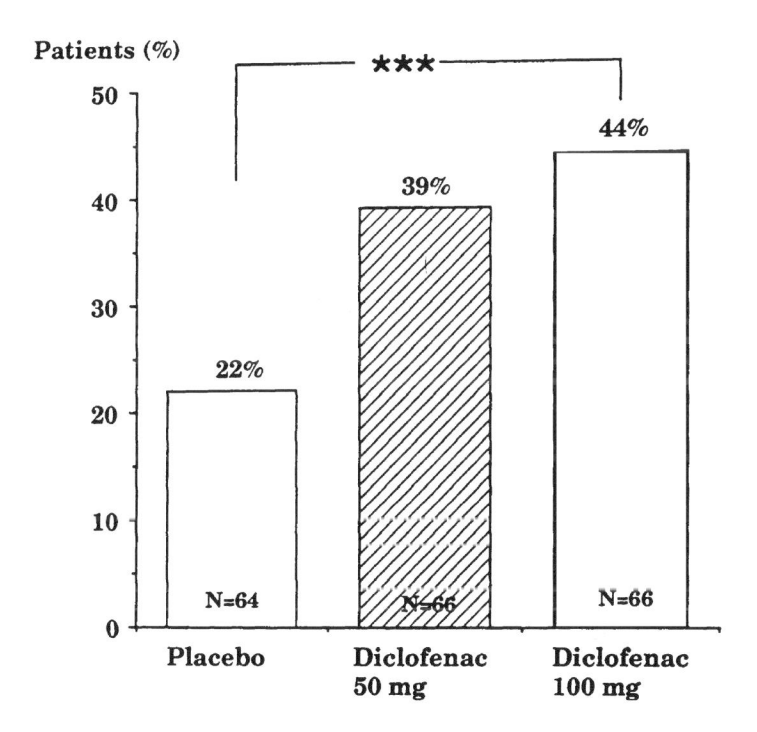

FIGURE 4.1 Efficacy of diclofenac, 50 and 100 mg by mouth, in the abortive treatment of migraine, defined as a reduction in headache intensity from moderate or severe to mild or no headache within *two* hours of treatment. From Dahlof C, Bjorkman R. Diclofenac-K (50 and 100 mg) and placebo in the acute treatment of migraine. Cephalalgia 1993; 13:117–123 with permission.

Indomethacin

Indomethacin (Indocid, UK; Indocin, US) was studied in a double-blind, placebo-controlled, *crossover* trial.[15] The trial involved 45 patients, 35 of whom completed the study. The dose of the medication was 100 mg by rectum, followed if necessary by 25 mg by mouth every four hours. With regard to overall efficacy, 63 percent of the patients responded better to indomethacin than to placebo and 11 percent responded better to placebo. With regard to adverse effects, six patients experienced an urge to defecate, three felt lightheaded, two spoke of burning in the rectum, and two complained of abdominal cramps. Indomethacin is not only a potent analgesic; it also mildly constricts the extracranial arteries in humans[16] and reduces neurogenic inflammation in the rat dura mater.[17]

Naproxen sodium

Naproxen sodium (Synflex, UK; Anaprox, US) was studied in a double-blind, placebo-controlled, *parallel* trial.[18] The trial involved 70 patients, 24 of whom completed the study. The dose of the medication was 825 mg by mouth, followed if necessary by 550 mg after one hour. When treated with naproxen sodium, the intensity of the headaches was 24 percent lower than treatment with placebo, and their duration was 20 percent shorter. Adverse effects were experienced more frequently with placebo than with the medication.

Naproxen sodium was compared with ergotamine in a double-blind, *parallel* study.[19] The trial involved 79 patients, 42 of whom completed the study. The dose of naproxen sodium was 750 mg by mouth, followed if necessary by two doses of 500 mg with intervals of a half hour. The dose of ergotamine was 2 mg by mouth, followed if necessary by two doses of 1 mg with intervals of a half hour. Fifty-four percent of the patients in the naproxen-sodium group experienced a good, very good or excellent response, as compared to 27 percent in the ergotamine group.

Naproxen sodium was compared with the combination of ergotamine and caffeine in a double-blind, placebo-controlled, *parallel* study.[20] The trial involved 161 patients, 122 of whom completed the study. The dose of naproxen sodium was 825 mg by mouth, followed if necessary by 275 mg after a half hour. The dose of ergotamine was 2 mg by mouth, followed if necessary by 1 mg after a half hour. In providing headache relief, naproxen sodium rather than ergotamine was significantly better than placebo, but naproxen sodium was *not* better than ergotamine.

Naproxen sodium was compared with the combination of ergotamine (2 mg), caffeine (91.5 mg), and cyclizine (50 mg) by mouth (Migwell, UK; not available in the US) in a double-blind, *parallel* study.[21] The trial involved 114 patients, 95 of whom completed the study. The dose of naproxen sodium was 825 mg by mouth, followed if necessary twice by 275 mg with intervals of a half hour. The ergotamine combination was also repeated twice if necessary in a dose of one-half tablet with intervals of a half hour. When taken within two hours of the onset of the headache, naproxen sodium decreased the intensity of the headaches by 31 percent, that of the nausea by 62 percent, and that of the photophobia by 45 percent. The ergotamine combination decreased the intensity of the headaches by 20 percent, that of the nausea by 43 percent, and that of the photophobia by 32 percent. Adverse effects were experienced by 28 percent of the patients in the naproxen-sodium group and by 41 percent in the ergotamine combination group. Stomach upset was the most common adverse effect in both treatment groups.

Tolfenamic acid

Tolfenamic acid (not available in the UK or US) was studied in a double-blind, placebo-controlled, *crossover* trial.[22] The trial involved 49 patients. The dose of the medication was 200 mg by mouth, repeated if necessary after one and a half hours. The duration of the headaches was 37 percent shorter when treated with tolfenamic acid than with placebo treatment. The addition of caffeine (200 or 300 mg) or metoclopramide (10 or 20 mg) did not increase the efficacy of the medication. Adverse effects were mild and were experienced by 10 percent of the patients.

Tolfenamic acid was compared with ergotamine in a double-blind, placebo-controlled, *crossover* study.[23] The trial involved 20 patients, all of whom completed the study. The dose of tolfenamic acid was 200 mg and of ergotamine 1 mg by mouth. The medications equally decreased the intensity and duration of the headaches. In comparison to placebo, the duration of the headaches was 55 percent shorter when treated with tolfenamic acid and 46 percent shorter when treated with ergotamine.

Narcotic Analgesics

Codeine and butorphanol are narcotic analgesics which were studied in the abortive treatment of migraine. *Codeine* was compared with aspirin in a double-blind, placebo-controlled, *crossover* trial.[5] The trial involved 259 patients, 198 of whom completed the study. The dose of the codeine was 25 mg by mouth, taken together with 400 mg acetaminophen. The dose of aspirin was 1,000 mg by mouth. Two hours after treatment, 50 percent of the patients obtained complete or almost complete relief of the headache with the combination of acetaminophen with codeine. With placebo treatment, 30 percent of the patients obtained this relief and with aspirin, 52 percent.

Butorphanol (not available in the UK; Stadol, US) was studied in two double-blind, placebo-controlled, *parallel* trials, administered by nasal spray. The spray contains 1 mg of the medication per insufflation. The first trial involved 63 patients, 32 of whom received the medication and 31 of whom received placebo.[24] The dose of butorphanol was 1 mg, repeated after one hour.

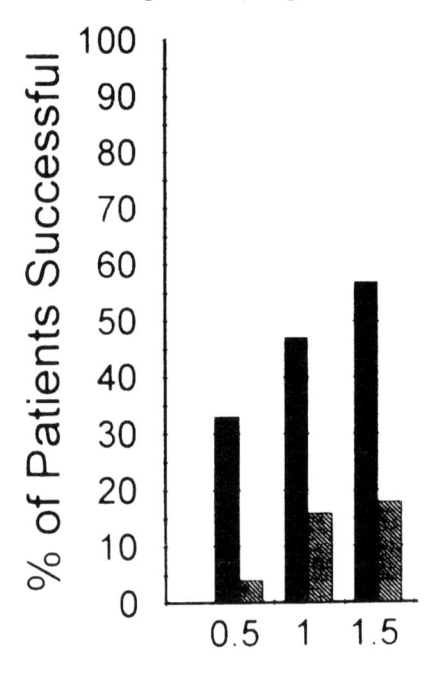

FIGURE 4.2 Efficacy of butorphanol, 1 or 2 mg by nasal spray, in the abortive treatment of migraine, defined as a reduction in headache intensity from moderate, severe or incapacitating to mild or no headache at 0.5, 1 and 1.5 hours after treatment. From Hoffert MJ, Couch JR, Diamond S, et al. Transnasal butorphanol in the treatment of acute migraine. Headache 1995; 35:65–69 with permission.

During the first three hours of treatment, the decrease in headache intensity was significantly better for those using butorphanol than for those using placebo. Adverse effects occurred in 91 percent of the patients in the butorphanol group and in 45 percent of those in the placebo group. The most common adverse effects were lightheadedness and drowsiness.

The second trial involved 157 patients, 107 of whom received butorphanol and 50 of whom received placebo.[25] The dose of the medication was 1 mg, if necessary repeated after 30 to 90 minutes. Efficacy was defined as a reduction in headache intensity from moderate, severe or incapacitating to mild or no headache. Within one hour of treatment, efficacy was obtained in 47 percent of the patients in the butorphanol group, as compared to 16 percent in the placebo group (Figure 4.2). With regard to adverse effects, 58 percent of the patients in the butorphanol group experienced lightheadedness, 38 percent complained of nausea or vomiting, and 29 percent felt drowsy as compared to 4, 18, and 0 percent, respectively, in the placebo group.

Vasoconstrictor Medications

The vasoconstrictor medications are divided into two groups: *sympathomimetic* and *serotoninergic vasoconstrictors.* The sympathomimetic vasoconstrictors release catecholamines from the sympathetic nerve terminals or directly stimulate the postsynaptic alpha-adrenergic receptors. The sympathomimetic vasoconstrictors are used mostly as decongestants (e.g., phenylephrine and phenylpropanolamine, directly and indirectly acting sympathomimetics, respectively).

In the United States, an indirectly acting sympathomimetic, *isometheptene*, is available for the abortive treatment of migraine. It is present in the combination preparation *Midrin*, which contains 65 mg isometheptene, 100 mg dichloralphenazone (a sedative), and 325 mg acetaminophen.

Isometheptene

Isometheptene was studied in a double-blind, placebo-controlled, *crossover* trial.[26] The trial involved 36 patients. The dose of the medication was 260 mg by mouth, taken at the onset of the headache, followed if necessary by 130 mg every one hour to a maximum of 780 mg. Isometheptene provided good or complete relief of the headaches in 42 percent, as compared to 29 percent with placebo treatment.

The combination of isometheptene, dichloralphenazone, and acetaminophen (i.e., Midrin), was also studied in a double-blind, placebo-controlled, *crossover* trial.[27] The trial involved 56 patients. The patients took two capsules at the onset of the headache, followed if necessary by one capsule every hour with a maximum of five. The combination provided significantly better relief of the headaches than did placebo.

Midrin was compared with the combination of ergotamine and caffeine in a double-blind, *crossover* trial.[28] The trial involved 38 patients. The patients took two capsules at the onset of the headache, followed if necessary by one capsule every hour with a maximum of six. The ergotamine-caffeine capsules contained 1 mg ergotamine and 100 mg caffeine. The intensity of the headaches was 15 percent lower with Midrin than with ergotamine and the nausea was 45 percent less.

As an indirectly acting sympathomimetic, isometheptene is contraindicated in patients treated with a monoamine oxidase inhibitor.

Scrotoninergic Vasoconstrictors

The serotoninergic vasoconstrictors are much more potent than the sympathomimetic vasoconstrictors. They are, therefore, contraindicated in patients with *hypertension* or *coronary artery disease* and those with significant risk factors for cardiovascular disease. The serotoninergic vasoconstrictors are ergotamine, dihydroergotamine, and sumatriptan. They supposedly induce vasoconstriction by stimulating serotonin-1 receptors. However, the extracranial arteries in humans do not contain serotonin-1 receptors but mostly contain serotonin-2 receptors.[29] The serotoninergic vasoconstrictors also reduce neurogenic inflammation, which is another mechanism involved in the pathogenesis of the migraine headache. This has been shown for ergotamine in humans (Figure 4.3)[30] and for dihydroergotamine[31] and sumatriptan[32] in the rat dura mater.

Ergotamine

Ergotamine (Gynergen, UK/US) is the oldest of the serotoninergic vasoconstrictors and was introduced in the treatment of migraine in 1926.[33] Figure 4.4 shows its potent vasoconstrictor effect on the superficial temporal artery in humans in relation to its effect on the migraine headache.[34] A summary of its reported efficacies in combination with caffine in the abortive treatment of migraine is presented in Table 4.5.

Ergotamine was studied in a double-blind, placebo-controlled, *crossover* trial.[35] The trial involved 88 patients, 79 of whom completed the study. The dose of the medication was 2 mg by mouth, followed if necessary by 1 mg after a half hour. Fifty-one percent of the patients obtained slight to considerable benefit from ergotamine and 58 percent from placebo. With regard to adverse effects, 15 percent of the patients experienced nausea from ergotamine and 4 percent got this result from placebo.

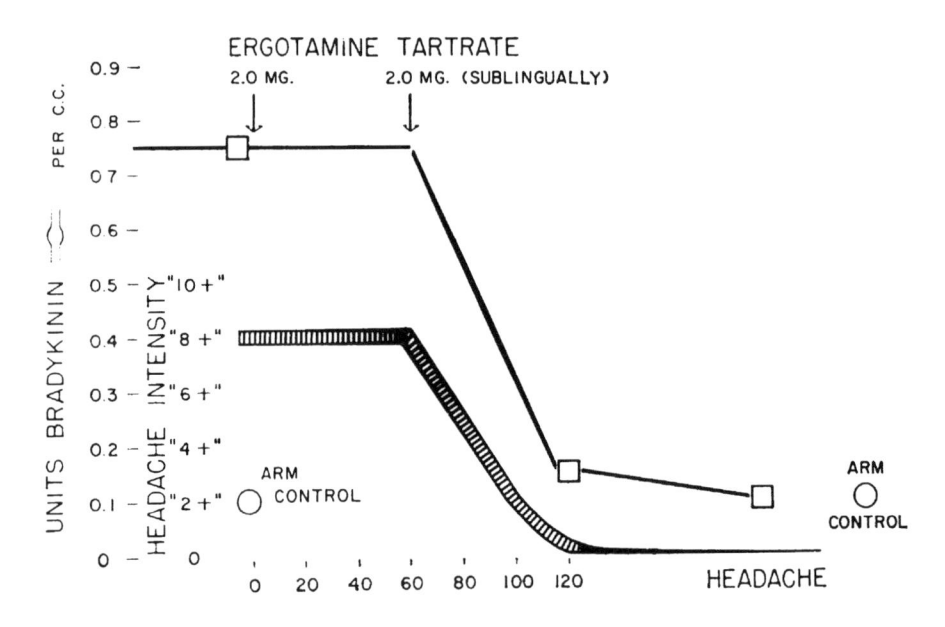

FIGURE 4.3 Effect of ergotamine, 4 mg by sublingual tablet, on the inflammatory activity of subcutaneous perfusates of the site of the migraine headache, measured in bradykinin units, in relation to the intensity of the pain. From Chapman LF, Ramos AO, Goodell H, et al. A humoral agent implicated in vascular headache of the migraine type. Arch Neurol 1960; 3:223–229 with permission.

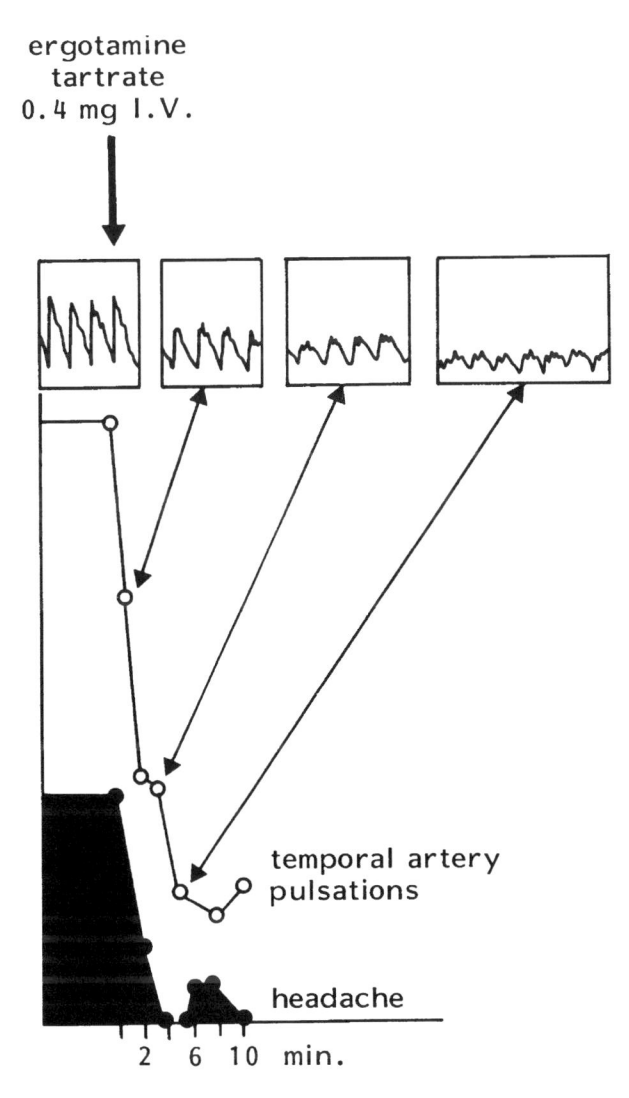

FIGURE 4.4 Effect of ergotamine, 0.4 mg by intravenous injection, on the pulsation amplitude of the superficial temporal artery in relation to the intensity of the migraine headache. From Graham JR, Wolff HG. Mechanism of migraine headache and action of ergotamine tartrate. Arch Neurol Psychiatry 1938; 39: 737–763 with permission.

Ergotamine is marketed in combination with caffeine as *Cafergot* (UK/US), which is available as a tablet *and* suppository. The combination with caffeine serves to increase the absorption of the medication.[36]

The Cafergot tablet contains 1 mg ergotamine and 100 mg caffeine and was studied in a double-blind, placebo-controlled, *parallel* trial.[37] The trial involved 307 patients, 254 of whom completed the study. The patients took two tablets at the onset of the headache, followed if necessary by one tablet every half hour with a maximum of six. Twenty-six percent of the patients in the Cafergot group obtained good to excellent results as compared to 10 percent in the placebo group. Adverse effects were experienced by 24 percent of the patients in the Cafergot group and by 4 percent in the placebo group.

TABLE 4.5
Reported efficacies of ergotamine-caffeine in the abortive treatment of migraine

Route	Efficacy	Study
Oral		
2 mg	48 percent efficacy* within 2 hours	Multinational Oral Sumatriptan and Cafergot Comparative Study Group, 1991[60]
2–6 mg	40 percent successfully treated	Blowers et al., 1981[38]
2–6 mg	26 percent good to excellent results	Friedman et al., 1989[37]
Rectal		
1–2 mg	73 percent complete relief within 3 hours	Graham, 1954[39]

*Defined as a reduction in headache intensity from moderate or severe to mild or no headache

The combination of ergotamine and caffeine was also studied in an *open* trial as an effervescent tablet (Effergot, UK; not available in the US).[38] The tablet contains 2 mg ergotamine and 50 mg caffeine and the patients took one tablet every half hour with a maximum of three. A total of 261 migraine headaches were treated in 68 patients, with a mean number of 2.25 tablets per headache. Forty percent of the headaches were successfully treated with the effervescent tablet and moderate relief was obtained in an additional 38 percent.

The Cafergot suppository contains 2 mg ergotamine and 100 mg caffeine. The combination of ergotamine and caffeine administered rectally was studied in an *open* trial of 100 patients during 577 headaches.[39] Seventy-three percent of the patients obtained complete relief of their migraine headaches within three hours of treatment and only five percent experienced adverse effects. The best results were obtained with suppositories containing 1 mg ergotamine and 100 mg caffeine, repeated if necessary after one hour.

Ergotamine administered rectally was studied in a double-blind, *crossover* trial in combination with metoclopramide to reduce the gastrointestinal adverse effects.[40] The dose of ergotamine was 1 or 2 mg; the metoclopramide dose was 20 mg. The best effects on the intensity and duration of the headaches and the occurrence of nausea were obtained with the suppository that contained 2 mg ergotamine and 20 mg metoclopramide.

Ergotamine was also studied by aerosol inhalation with each insufflation containing 0.36 mg of the medication (Medihaler-Ergotamine, UK; not available in the US). In an *open* study of 46 patients, 83 percent obtained excellent relief of their headaches.[41] In another *open* study of 48 patients, 58 percent obtained complete relief of their headaches within a half hour of treatment.[42] In general, one to three insufflations were required to obtain these results. Adverse effects, mostly nausea or vomiting, were experienced by 10 to 20 percent of patients.

Dihydroergotamine

Dihydroergotamine (Dihydergot, UK; DHE 45, US), a derivative of ergotamine, was introduced in the treatment of migraine in 1945.[43] Its pharmacology is very similar to that of ergotamine with quantitative rather than qualitative differences.[44] As it is about four times less potent as a vasoconstrictor but ten times less potent as an emetic, it is generally better tolerated than ergotamine with less nausea and vomiting. The vasoconstrictor effect of dihydroergotamine on the superficial temporal artery in humans is shown in Figure 4.5. A summary of its reported efficacies in the abortive treatment of migraine is presented in Table 4.6.

Dihydroergotamine was studied in four double-blind, placebo-controlled, trials, administered by nasal spray (Migramist; not available in the UK or US). The spray contains 0.5 mg of the medication per insufflation. The first was a *crossover* trial and involved 17 patients, 15 of whom completed the study.[45] The dose of the medication was 0.5 mg every half hour with a maximum of 1.5 mg. The overall efficacy of dihydroergotamine was rated by the patients as 52 percent, compared to 43 percent for placebo.

The second was also a *crossover* trial and involved 112 patients, 100 of whom completed the study.[46] The dose of the medication was 1 mg which was repeated after 15 minutes. Four hours after treatment, headache intensity was decreased from baseline by an average of one point on a four-point scale (mild, moderate, severe, and incapacitating) (Figure 4.6).

The third and fourth were *parallel* trials and involved 229 patients, 206 of whom completed the study.[47] The dose of the medication was 1 mg, which was repeated after 15 minutes. Four hours after treatment, the reduction in headache intensity was 0.65 mg and 1.06, repectively, for the headaches treated with dihydroergotamine and 0.04 and 0.01, respectively, for those treated with placebo. Headache intensity was rated on the same four-point scale as mentioned above. The majority of the adverse effects reported by the patients treated with dihydroergotamine were nasopharyngeal (nasal congestion, throat discomfort, and nasal irritation).

Dihydroergotamine was also studied in a double-blind, placebo-controlled, *crossover* trial, administered by intravenous injection.[48] The trial involved 37 patients. They were first treated with prochlorperazine (Stemetil, UK; Compazine, US), 5 mg intravenously. The dihydroergotamine was administered a half hour *after* the prochlorperazine in a dose of 0.75 mg. The prochlorperazine reduced the intensity of the headaches by 37 percent. Subsequent administration of dihydroergotamine further reduced the intensity

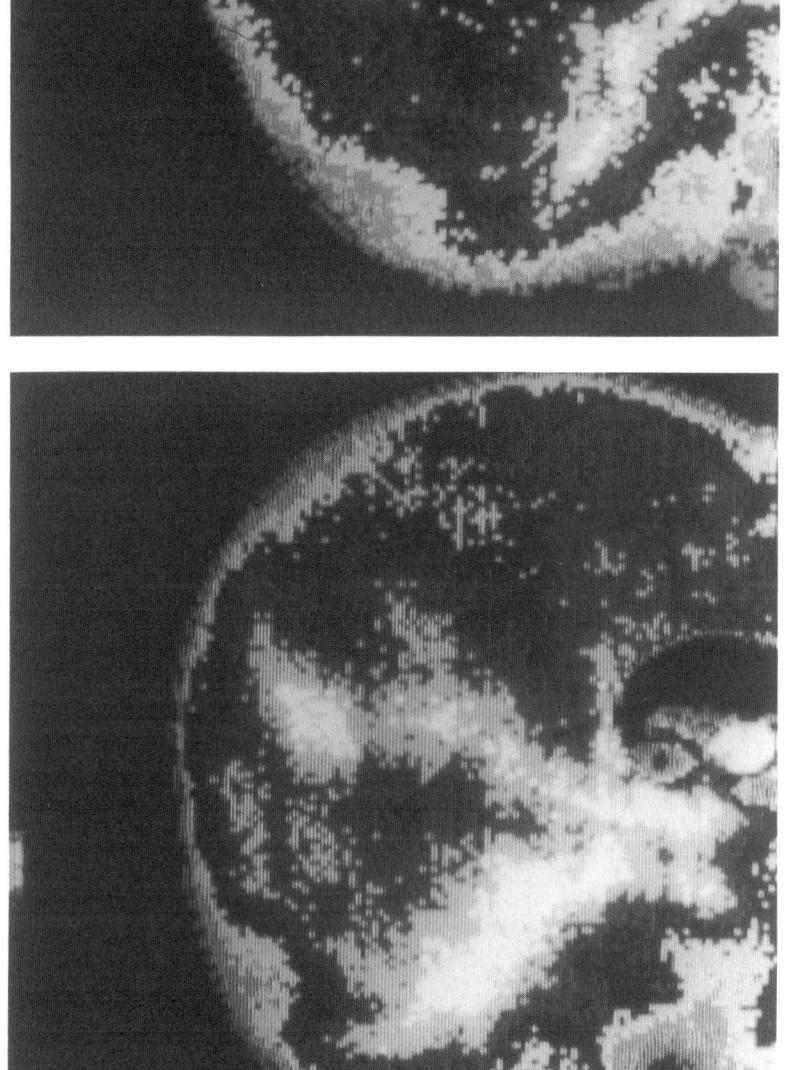

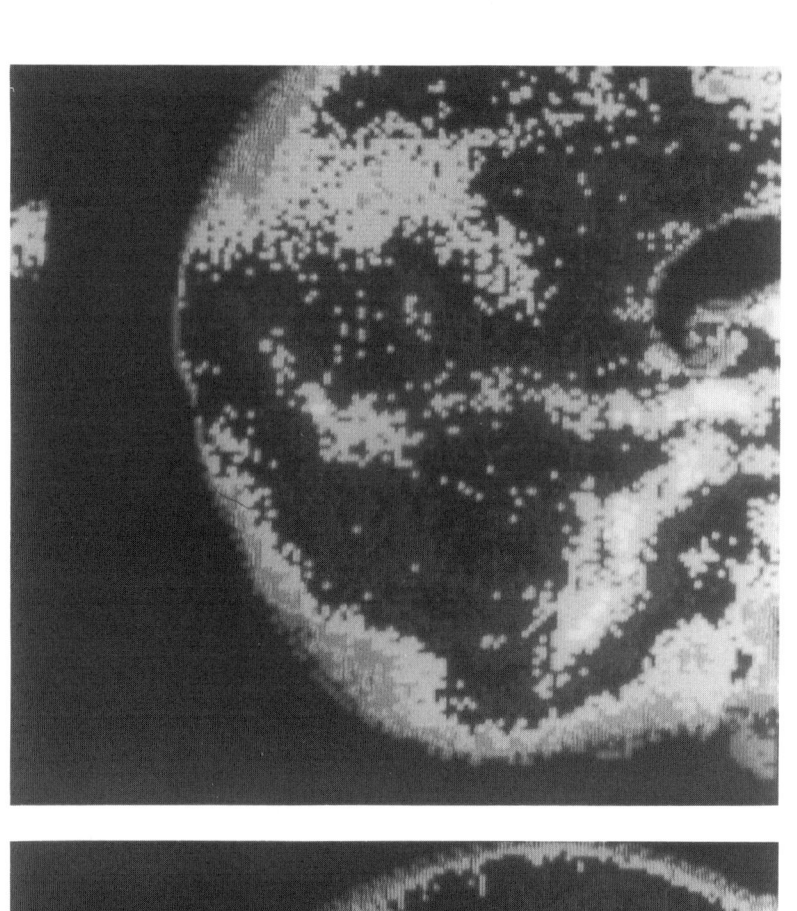

FIGURE 4.5 Thermography of the lateral side of the head, showing the superficial temporal artery in white, before (left) and 30 minutes after administration of 0.5 mg dihydroergotamine intravenously (right).

TABLE 4.6
Reported efficacies of dihydroergotamine in the abortive treatment of migraine

Route	Efficacy	Study
Nasal		
0.5–1.5 mg	52 percent overall efficacy*	Tulunay et al., 1987[45]
Intramuscular		
1 mg	85 percent very marked or complete relief	Hartman, 1945[51]
1 mg	60 percent complete relief within 4 hours	Saadah, 1992[50]
Intravenous		
1–2 mg	37 percent decrease in headache intensity within 1 hour	Bell et al., 1990[52]
1 mg with 10 mg metoclopramide	86 percent pain relief within 1 hour	Scherl & Wilson, 1995[49]
1 mg with 10 mg metoclopramide	70 percent decrease in headache intensity within 1 hour	Belgrade et al., 1989[53]
0.75 mg with 5 mg prochlorperazine	60 percent reduction in headache intensity within 1 hour	Callaham & Raskin, 1986[48]

*Based on patient rating.

of the headaches within one hour by 60 percent, as compared to 25 percent with placebo. Nausea occurred as an adverse effect of the medication in 37 percent of the patients.

Dihydroergotamine administered intravenously with metoclopramide was compared with the combination of *meperidine* (Pethidine, UK; Demerol, US) with promethazine intramuscularly in a double-blind *parallel* study.[49] The trial involved 27 patients, all of whom completed the study. The dose of dihydroergotamine was 0.5 mg, given with 10 mg metoclopramide; the meperidine dose was 75 mg, given with 25 mg promethazine. One hour after treatment, pain relief was 86 percent in the patients treated with dihydroergotamine/metoclopramide and 77 percent in those treated with meperidine/promethazine. Adverse effects, in particular lightheadedness and drowsiness, were more common in the meperidine/promethazine than in the dihydroergotamine/metoclopramide group.

Dihydroergotamine was studied in several *open* trials, administered by intramuscular or intravenous injection. Administered intramuscularly, in a study of 43 patients, 1 mg of the medication provided complete relief in over

44   *Management of Migraine*

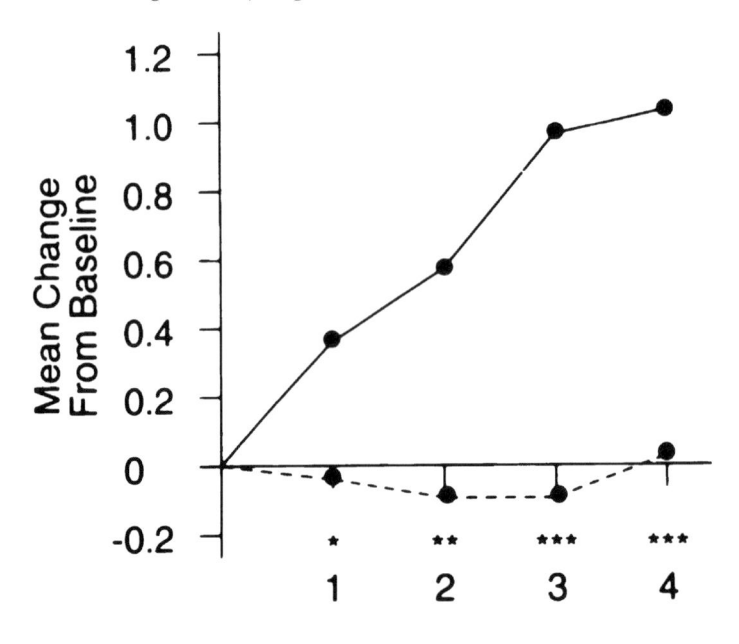

FIGURE 4.6   Effect of dihydroergotamine, 2 mg by nasal spray, on headache intensity, defined as mild, moderate, severe or incapacitating, during the first four hours after treatment. From Ziegler D, Ford R, Kriegler J, et al. Dihydroergotamine nasal spray for the acute treatment of migraine. Neurology 1994; 44:447–453 with permission.

60 percent of headaches within four hours of treatment (Figure 4.7).[50] In another study of 20 patients, 1 mg dihydroergotamine provided very marked or complete relief of headaches in 85 percent.[51] In the first study, 24 percent of the patients experienced nausea, and in the second it was experienced by 5 percent.

Administered intravenously, in a study of 26 patients, 1 or 2 mg of the medication decreased the intensity of the headaches by 37 percent within one hour of treatment.[52] In another study of 21 patients, 1 mg dihydroergotamine in combination with 10 mg metoclopramide decreased the intensity of the headaches by 70 percent within one hour of treatment.[53]

Sumatriptan

Sumatriptan (Imigran, UK; Imitrex, US), a derivative of serotonin, was introduced in the treatment of migraine in 1988.[54] Its potent vasoconstrictor effect on the human meningeal, cerebral, and temporal arteries is shown in Figure 4.8.[55] Sumatriptan is much more selective in its receptor interactions than the ergot medications, ergotamine and dihydroergotamine, as is shown

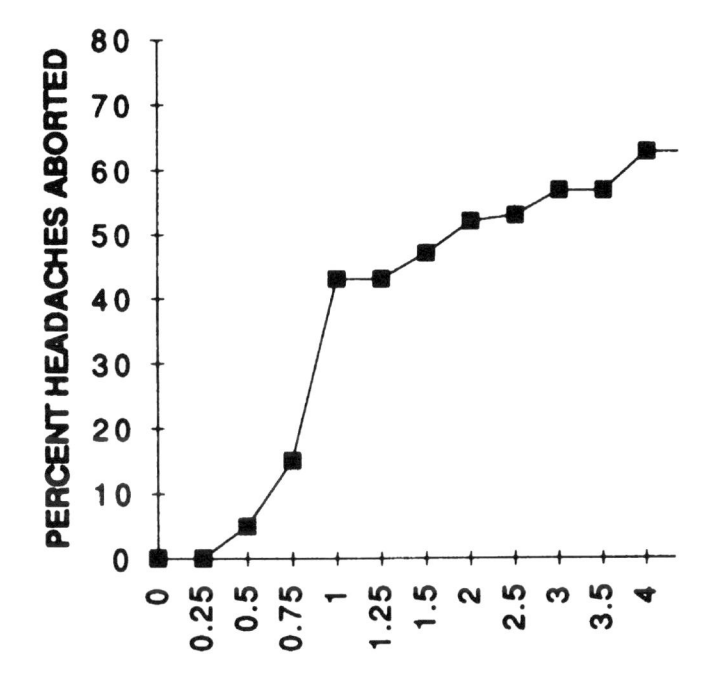

FIGURE 4.7 Efficacy of dihydroergotamine, 1 mg by intramuscular injection, in the abortive treatment of migraine, defined as the percentage of headaches aborted. From Saadah HA. Abortive headache therapy with intramuscular dihydroergotamine. Headache 1992; 32:18–20 with permission.

in Table 4.7.[56] It has affinity only for the serotonin-1A and -1D receptors, whereas the ergot medications have affinity for the serotonin-1 and -2 receptors, as well as for the alpha-1 and -2 receptors and for the dopamine-2 receptors. An intriguing fact about sumatriptan is that it potently constricts the human temporal artery though the artery is virtually devoid of serotonin-1 receptors.[29] A summary of its reported efficacies in the abortive treatment of migraine is presented in Table 4.8.

Sumatriptan, when administered orally, has the best ratio of efficacy to safety in a dose of 100 mg. In the double-blind, placebo-controlled, *parallel* dose-finding study involving 1,130 patients, the efficacy of the medication was 67 percent, as compared to 27 percent with placebo (Figure 4.9).[57] Efficacy was defined as a reduction in headache intensity from moderate or severe to mild or no headache within *two* hours of treatment. Adverse effects were experienced by 36 percent of the patients in the sumatriptan group and by 17 percent in the placebo group. The most common adverse effects were nausea, vomiting, fatigue, lightheadedness, bad taste, numbness, and weakness.

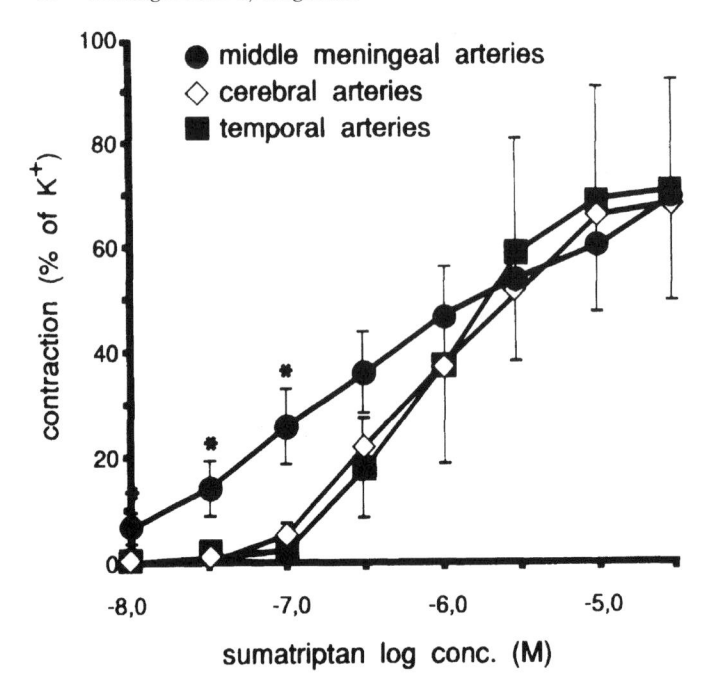

FIGURE 4.8 Effect of sumatriptan on the human meningeal, cerebral, and temporal arteries. From Jansen I, Edvinsson L, Mortensen A, Olesen J. Sumatriptan is a potent vasoconstrictor of human dural arteries via a 5-HT$_1$-like receptor. Cephalalgia 1992; 12:202–205 with permission.

TABLE 4.7
Affinities (K$_i$) of dihydroergotamine and sumatriptan for the serotoninergic, adrenergic, and dopaminergic receptors

	Dihydroergotamine	Sumatriptan
Serotonin-1A	1.2	100
Serotonin-1C	39	>10,000
Serotonin-1D	19	17
Serotonin-2	78	>10,000
Serotonin-3	>10,000	>10,000
Alpha-1	6.6	>10,000
Alpha-2	3.4	>10,000
Beta	960	>10,000
Dopamine-1	700	>10,000
Dopamine-2	98	>10,000

Adapted from McCarthy BG, Peroutka SJ, 1989 with permission.[56]

TABLE 4.8
Reported efficacies of sumatriptan in the abortive treatment of migraine

Route	Efficacy	Study
Oral		
100 mg	67 percent efficacy* within 2 hours	Oral Sumatriptan Dose-Defining Study Group, 1991[57]
100 mg	66 percent efficacy* within 2 hours	Multinational Oral Sumatriptan and Cafergot Comparative Study Group, 1991[60]
100 mg	56–65 percent efficacy* within 2 hours	Oral Sumatriptan and Aspirin plus Metoclopramide Comparative Study Group, 1992[59]
100 mg	55 percent efficacy* within 2 hours	Ferrari et al., 1994[58]
100–200 mg	73 percent efficacy* within 4 hours	Ferrari et al., 1994[58]
Nasal		
40 mg	75 percent efficacy* within 2 hours	Finnish Sumatriptan Group, 1991[61]
Subcutaneous		
6 mg	70 percent efficacy* within 1 hour	Cady et al., 1991[62]
6–12 mg	81 percent efficacy* within 2 hours	Cady et al., 1994[62]
6 mg	75 percent efficacy* within 2 hours	Subcutaneous Sumatriptan International Study Group, 1991[63]
12 mg	81 percent efficacy* within 2 hours	Subcutaneous Sumatriptan International Study Group, 1991[63]
6 mg	77 percent efficacy* within 1 hour	Sumatriptan Auto Injector Study Group, 1991[64]
6 mg	56 percent efficacy* within 1 hour	Russell et al., 1994[66]

*Defined as a reduction in headache intensity from moderate or severe to mild or no headache.

48   *Management of Migraine*

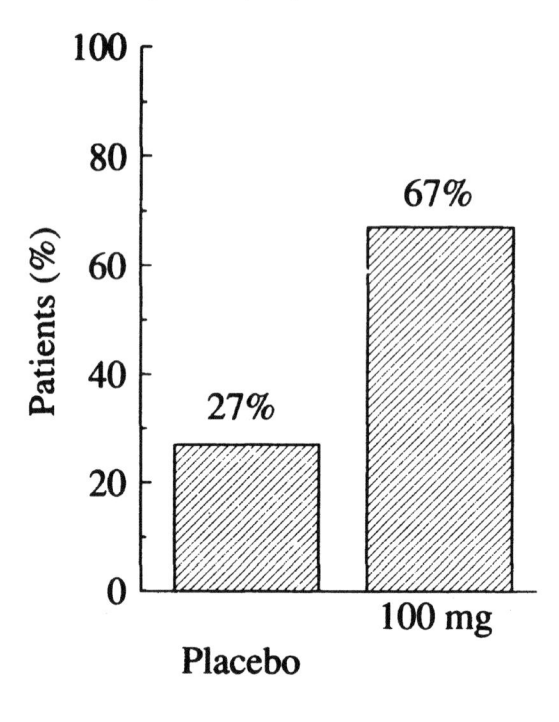

FIGURE 4.9 Efficacy of sumatriptan, 100 mg by mouth, in the abortive treatment of migraine, defined as a reduction in headache intensity from moderate or severe to mild or no headache within two hours of treatment. From the Oral Sumatriptan Dose-Defining Study Group. Sumatriptan—an oral dose-defining study. Eur Neurol 1991; 31: 300–305 with permission.

A second study of sumatriptan, administered in a dose of 100 mg by mouth, involved 1,449 patients, 1,086 of whom completed the trial.[58] Efficacy was again defined as a reduction in headache intensity from moderate or severe to mild or no headache. Two hours after treatment, 55 percent of the patients had achieved this level of efficacy. Four hours after treatment, 73 percent had achieved this efficacy, whether or not a second dose of the medication was taken after two hours. Of the 793 patients who had achieved the above level of efficacy after four hours, 24 percent experienced a recurrence of moderate or severe headache within 24 hours of treatment. Sumatriptan, 100 mg by mouth, administered at that point again provided relief of headache as defined previously in 70 percent of the patients, as compared to 38 percent with placebo. Adverse effects were experienced by up to 35 percent of the patients. The most common adverse effects were nausea, vomiting, heaviness, lightheadedness, drowsiness, and fatigue.

Sumatriptan was compared with aspirin plus metoclopramide in a double-blind, placebo-controlled, *parallel* study.[59] The dose of sumatriptan was 100 mg by mouth; the aspirin plus metoclopramide dose was 900 plus 10 mg by mouth. The trial involved 382 patients, 355 of whom completed the study. Sumatriptan was more effective than aspirin plus metoclopramide, with efficacies of 56 to 65 percent and 34 to 45 percent, respectively. Efficacy was defined as before (i.e., a reduction in headache intensity from moderate or severe to mild or no headache within two hours of treatment). Relief from nausea, vomiting, photo- and phonophobia was similar in the two treatment groups. Adverse effects were experienced by 42 percent of the patients in the sumatriptan group and by 29 percent in the aspirin-plus-metoclopramide group. The most common adverse effects in both groups were nausea or vomiting and fatigue.

Sumatriptan was also compared with Cafergot in a double-blind, *parallel* study.[60] The dose of sumatriptan was 100 mg by mouth; the Cafergot dose was two tablets (i.e., 2 mg ergotamine plus 200 mg caffeine). The trial involved 580 patients, 577 of whom completed the study. Sumatriptan was more effective than Cafergot, with efficacies of 66 and 48 percent, respectively (Figure 4.10). Efficacy was again defined as a reduction in headache intensity from moderate or severe to mild or no headache within *two* hours of treatment. Adverse effects were experienced by 45 percent of the patients in the sumatriptan group and by 39 percent in the Cafergot group. The most common adverse effects of sumatriptan were bad taste, followed by fatigue, nausea, and vomiting; Cafergot most commonly produced adverse effects of nausea and vomiting.

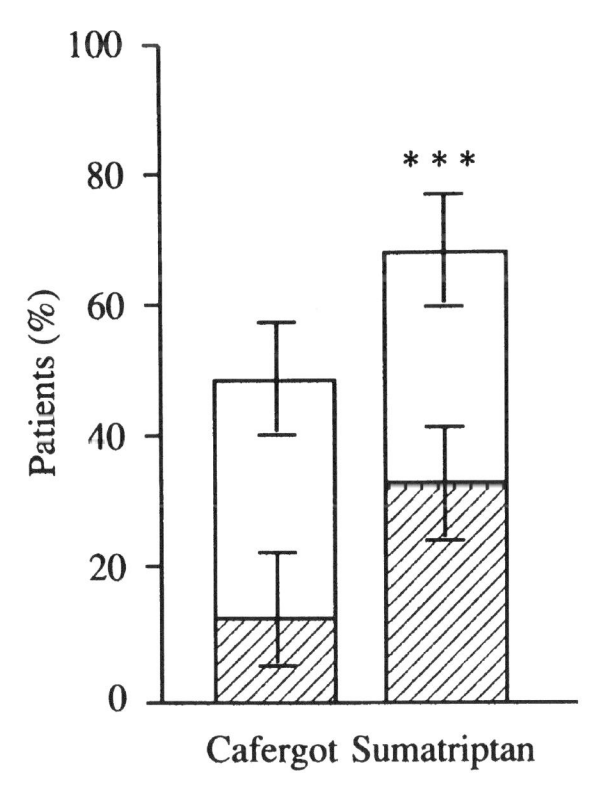

FIGURE 4.10 Efficacy of sumatriptan, 100 mg by mouth, or Cafergot, two tablets (i.e., 2 mg ergotamine plus 200 mg caffeine) in the abortive treatment of migraine, defined as a reduction in headache intensity from moderate or severe to mild or no headache within two hours of treatment. From the Multinational Oral Sumatriptan and Cafergot Comparative Study Group. A randomized, double-blind comparison of sumatriptan and Cafergot in the acute treatment of migraine. Eur Neurol 1991; 31: 314–322 with permission.

Sumatriptan was studied in a double-blind, placebo-controlled, *parallel* trial, administered by intranasal spray (not available in the UK or US).[61] The spray contains 20 mg of the medication per insufflation. The trial involved 76 patients, 73 of whom completed the study. The dose of the medication was 20 mg, which was repeated after 15 minutes. The efficacy of sumatriptan was 75 percent, as compared to 32 percent with placebo. Efficacy was again defined as a reduction in headache intensity from moderate or severe to mild or no headache within *two* hours of treatment. Adverse effects were experienced by 46 percent of the patients in the sumatriptan group and by 14 percent in the placebo group.

Sumatriptan was studied in two double-blind, placebo-controlled, *parallel* trials, administered by subcutaneous injection in a dose of 6 mg. The first study involved 1,104 patients, 734 of whom received sumatriptan and 370 of whom received placebo.[62] Efficacy was defined as a reduction in headache intensity from moderate or severe to mild or no headache within *one* hour of treatment. Sumatriptan achieved this level of efficacy in 70 percent of the patients as compared to 22 percent with placebo. Two hours after treatment, the efficacy of the medication was 81 percent, compared to 34 percent with placebo, whether or not a second dose of sumatriptan was given after one hour. The medication also significantly reduced the nausea and photophobia associated with the headaches. The most common adverse effects were injection-site reactions, tingling, lightheadedness, warm-hot sensation, burning, and heaviness or pressure.

The second study involved 527 patients, 422 of whom received sumatriptan and 105 of whom received placebo.[63] Two hours after treatment, efficacy as earlier defined was achieved by 75 percent of the patients who had received one injection of the medication, by 81 percent of those who had received two injections with a one-hour interval, and by 30 percent of those who had received two placebo injections. Sumatriptan was also significantly more effective than placebo in relieving nausea, vomiting, photo- and phonophobia. The most common adverse effects were injection-site reactions, heaviness, warm-hot sensation, and pressure.

Sumatriptan was also studied in two double-blind, placebo-controlled trials, administered by subcutaneous injection in a dose of 6 mg with the use of an auto-injector. The first was a *parallel* trial and involved 264 patients, 235 of whom completed the study.[64] The efficacy of sumatriptan was 77 percent, as compared to 26 percent with placebo (Figure 4.11). Efficacy was defined as a reduction in headache intensity from moderate or severe to mild or no headache within *one* hour of treatment. Adverse effects were experienced by 39 percent of the patients in the sumatriptan group and by 19 percent in the placebo group. The adverse effects were mostly injection-site reactions, followed by flushing, lightheadedness, nausea, vomiting, and neck tightness.

The second was a *crossover* trial and involved 230 patients, 209 of whom completed the study.[65] One hour after treatment, efficacy as defined

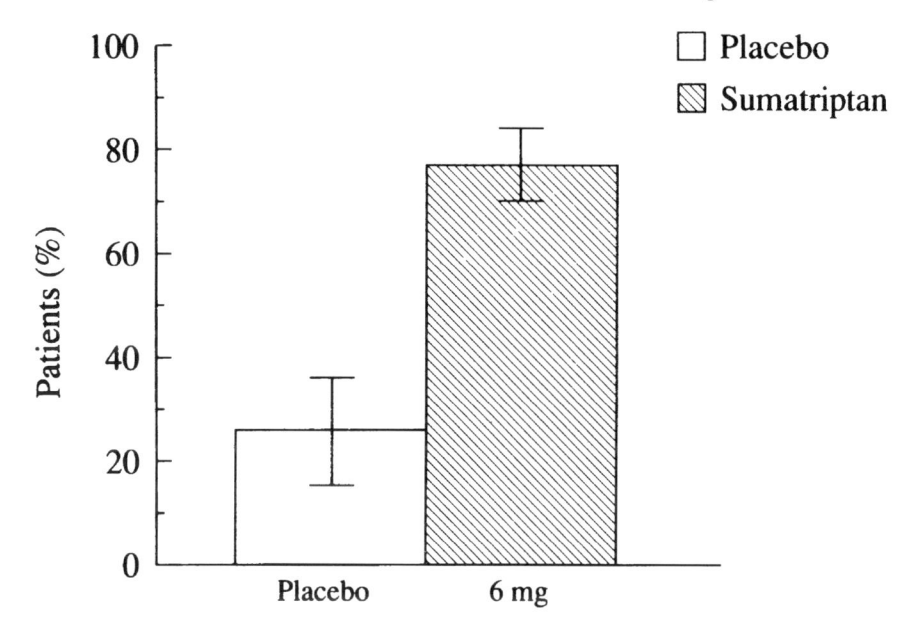

FIGURE 4.11 Efficacy of sumatriptan, 6 mg by subcutaneous injection with the use of an auto-injector, in the abortive treatment of migraine, defined as a reduction in headache intensity from moderate or severe to mild or no headache within one hour of treatment. From the Sumatriptan Auto-Injector Study Group. Self-treatment of acute migraine with subcutaneous sumatriptan using an auto-injector device. Eur Neurol 1991; 31:323–331 with permission.

above was achieved in 56 percent of the headaches treated with sumatriptan and in 8 percent of those treated with placebo. Resolution of nausea, photo- and phonophobia was also more comon in the headaches treated with sumatriptan than in those treated with placebo. Adverse effects occurred in 34 percent after treatment with sumatriptan and in 2 percent after placebo treatment.

The auto-injector was also used in a double-blind, placebo-controlled, *parallel* study of the effect of sumatriptan on the migraine aura.[66] The trial involved 153 patients, 80 of whom received 6 mg sumatriptan subcutaneously and 73 of whom received placebo at the start of or during the aura. The median duration of the aura was 25 minutes in the sumatriptan group and 30 minutes in the placebo group. Within six hours of treatment, 68 percent of the patients in the sumatriptan group and 75 percent of those in the placebo group developed a moderate or severe headache.

Efficacy

With regard to the *efficacy* of the abortive antimigraine medications, a summary of rounded estimates is presented in Table 4.9. When compared with placebo, the estimated efficacies are based on an assumed placebo response of 20 percent. The simple analgesics (aspirin, acetaminophen, and ibuprofen) have an estimated efficacy of 50 percent. The addition of a gastrokinetic medication (e.g., domperidone or metoclopramide) increases the efficacy of the simple analgesics to 60 percent. The nonsteroidal anti-inflammatory analgesics also have an estimated efficacy of 60 percent. Codeine with acetaminophen and butorphanol by nasal spray have estimated efficacies of 50 percent. Isometheptene, the sympathomimetic vasoconstrictor present in Midrin, has a similar efficacy of 50 percent. The combination of ergotamine and caffeine in the Cafergot tablet has an efficacy of 40 percent, whereas the Cafergot suppository has an estimated efficacy of 70 percent. Dihydroergotamine by nasal spray has an efficacy of 50 percent, whereas the intramuscular injection has an estimated efficacy of 70 percent and the intravenous injection of 60 percent. The sumatriptan 100 mg tablet has an estimated efficacy of 65 percent, the nasal spray of 75 percent, and the 6 mg subcutaneous injection has an 80 percent efficacy.

In general, the medications provide the estimated relief within one to three hours of treatment. The slowest relief is obtained with administration by mouth, partially because of the abnormal functioning of the gastrointes-

TABLE 4.9
Abortive antimigraine medications with rounded estimates of their efficacy

Analgesic	*Efficacy*
Simple analgesics	50 percent
Simple analgesic plus gastrokinetic	60 percent
Nonsteroidal anti-inflammatory analgesics	60 percent
Codeine plus acetaminophen-butorphanol nasal spray	50 percent
Isometheptene (Midrin)	50 percent
Ergotamine plus caffeine	
Tablet	40 percent
Suppository	70 percent
Dihydroergotamine	
Nasal spray	50 percent
Intramuscular injection	70 percent
Intravenous injection	60 percent
Sumatriptan	
Tablet	65 percent
Nasal spray	75 percent
Subcutaneous injection	80 percent

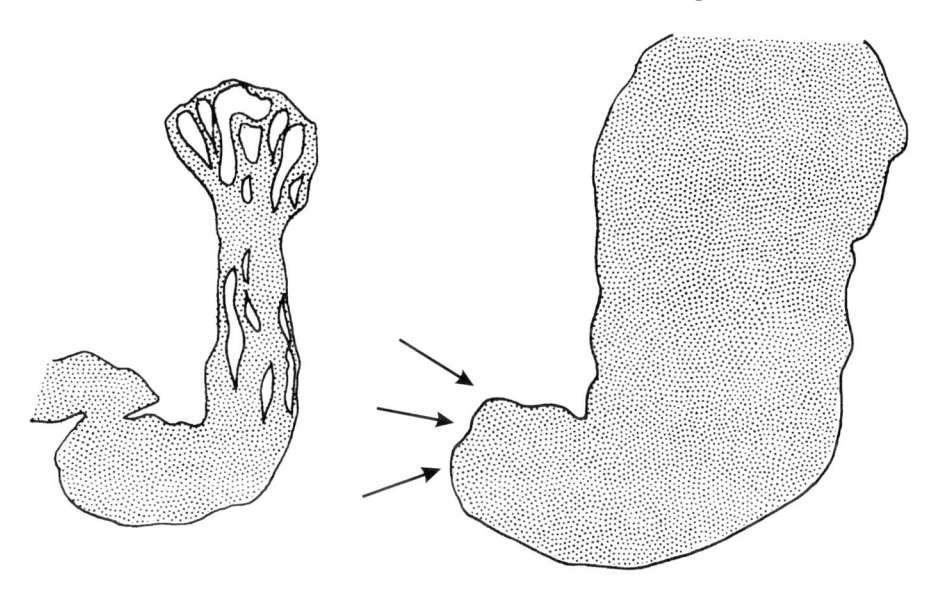

FIGURE 4.12 Upper gastrointestinal tract during a migraine attack (right) and between attacks (left), showing atony and dilation of the stomach with closure of the pyloric sphincter (arrows) during the attack. Adapted from Kaufman J, Levine I. Acute gastric dilatation of the stomach during attack of migraine. Radiology 1936; 27:301–302.

tinal tract. This abnormal functioning results in atony and dilation of the stomach with closure of the pyloric sphincter (Figure 4.12).[67] It is associated with a delay in gastric emptying, which correlates with the intensity of the headache, nausea, and photophobia.[68] The abnormal functioning also decreases the absorption of oral medications which was demonstrated for aspirin (Figure 4.13),[69] acetaminophen,[70] naproxen,[71] and tolfenamic acid.[72] The impaired absorption correlates with the intensity of the headache and nausea but *not* with the duration of the headache or the type of migraine.[73]

Metoclopramide, 20 mg by rectum or 10 mg by intramuscular injection, improves the impaired absorption of the oral medications (Figure 4.13).[69] In a study it also increased the efficacy of acetaminophen[12] and the same is true for domperidone which, like metoclopramide, is a gastrokinetic antiemetic.[11]

Duration of Action

With regard to the *adverse effects*, the simple analgesics probably are tolerated best, followed by the nonsteroidal anti-inflammatory analgesics. The isometheptene combination Midrin generally is well-tolerated also, though

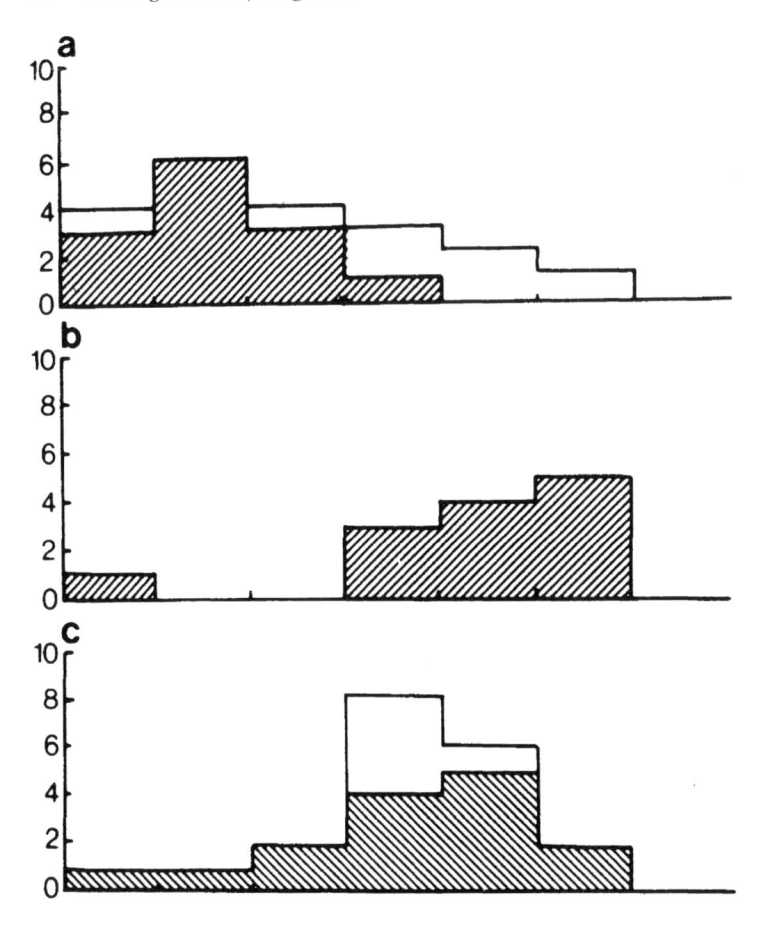

FIGURE 4.13 Distribution of the plasma salicylate level, 30 minutes after ingestion of 900 mg effervescent aspirin. A=during the migraine attack; B=in control subjects; C=during the migraine attack but *after* administration of 10 mg metoclopramide by intramuscular injection. From Volans GN. The effect of metoclopramide on the absorption of effervescent aspirin in migraine. Br J Clin Pharmacol 1975; 2:57–63 with permission.

it sometimes causes drowsiness. Codeine often causes nausea and constipation, whereas butorphanol often causes orthostatic hypotension. Ergotamine and dihydroergotamine are notorious for causing nausea and vomiting and also can cause leg cramps. Sumatriptan also causes nausea and vomiting but to a much lesser extent than the ergot medications. It can also cause flushing, numbness, and tightness, especially of the upper chest, anterior neck, and face.

With regard to their *duration of action*, the medications are all relatively short-acting except for the ergot medications. Therefore, the headache may return when the effect of the medication wears off. This has been particularly well studied for sumatriptan, which has a plasma half-life of two hours. Therefore, the medication is eliminated from the plasma in ten hours, and the headache returns within 24 hours of treatment in 40 to 60 percent of cases. Ergotamine is also eliminated from the plasma in ten hours but causes vasoconstriction for at least three days (Figure 4.14).[74] This discrepancy between plasma level and vasoconstrictor effect is caused by the very strong binding of the medication to the serotonin receptors. Ergotamine binds to the receptors 100 times more strongly than serotonin, the receptors' own biological substrate.[75] Therefore, it may provide much longer lasting relief of the headache, and the same is true for dihydroergotamine. This is also suggested by the lower recurrence of headache in the previously mentioned comparative study of sumatriptan and Cafergot.[60] In this study, the recurrence of headache within 24 hours of treatment was 41 percent in the sumatriptan group and 30 percent in the Cafergot group.

The negative side of the longer duration of action of the ergot medications is that they cannot be used frequently and, probably, should not be used more often than once per week. Otherwise, a gradual increase in frequency of the headaches occurs, sometimes to the extent of daily occurrence. This is due to the development of a vicious cycle in which the decrease in the effect of the vasoconstrictor medication is followed by rebound vasodilation and the occurrence of another headache. Patients in such a rebound cycle do *not* respond to preventive medications and have to be withdrawn from the offending vasoconstrictor. When this vasoconstrictor is an ergot medication, the withdrawal is generally associated with severe headache, nausea, and vomiting. The withdrawal lasts from one to seven days, but the improvement is often dramatic. In a study of 30 patients who were successfully withdrawn, 20 experienced a more than 50 percent reduction in headache days.[76] Unfortunately, the relapse rate is high, and in the same study, 10 of the 40 initially withdrawn patients went back to taking the ergot medication.

Choice of Treatment

The choice of abortive treatment depends in particular on two features of the headaches: their time of onset and their duration. With regard to the time of onset, migraine headaches either come about during the day, or are present on awakening in the morning or wake the patient at night. When they come about during the day, they generally build up in intensity over one to several hours, allowing relatively early treatment. With early treatment, it is possible to use oral medications that are no longer absorbed when the headache has progressed. When the headache is present on awakening in the morning or wakes the patient at night, the functioning of the gastrointestinal tract is already disturbed to the extent that the absorption of oral medications is impaired.

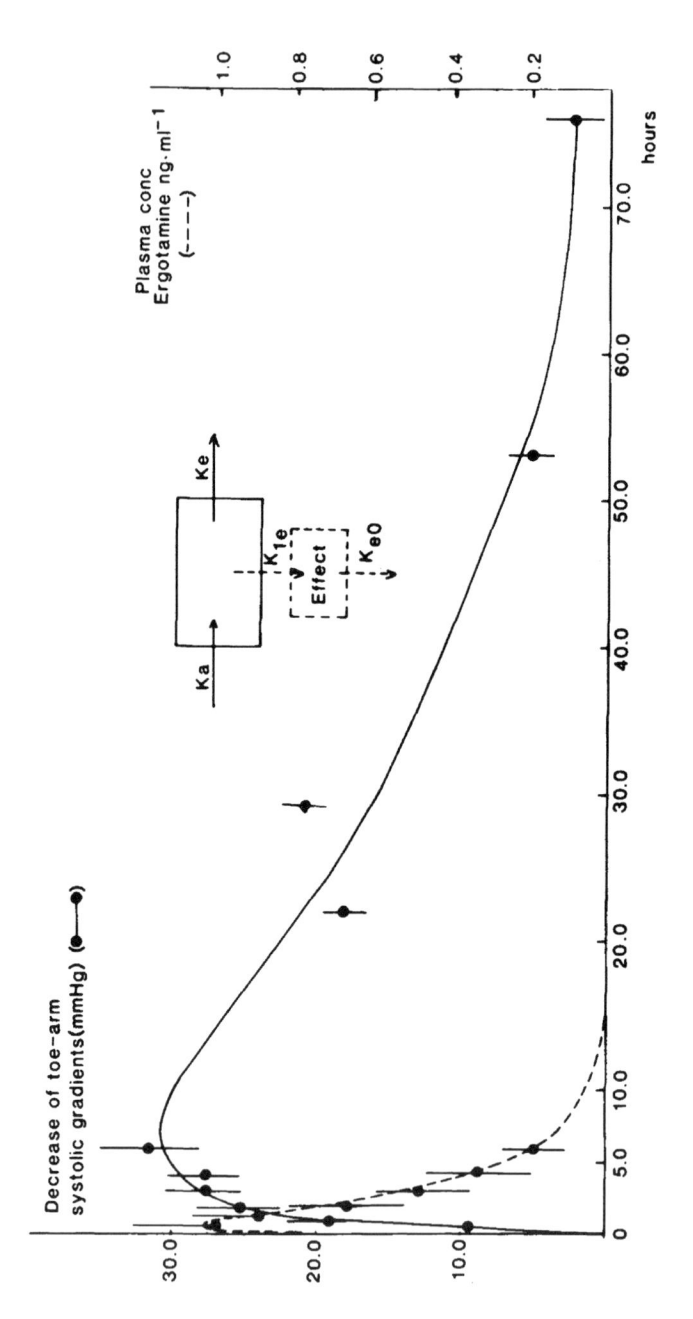

FIGURE 4.14 Ergotamine plasma level (interrupted line) and vasoconstrictor effect. expressed as a decrease in toe-arm systolic gradient (solid line), after administration of 0.5 mg ergotamine intramuscularly. From Tfelt-Hansen P, Paalzow L. Intramuscular ergotamine: Plasma levels and dynamic activity. Clin Pharmacol Ther 1985; 37:29–35 with permission.

When the headache comes about during the day, treatment should be initiated with a gastrokinetic medication (e.g., domperidone or metoclopramide). Both medications are available in tablets of 10 mg, and the usual doses are 20 mg for domperidone and 10 mg for metoclopramide. The medications do *not* cause drowsiness and are also otherwise generally well-tolerated. In classic migraine or migraine with aura, the medications can be taken during the aura.

Initiation of the headache treatment should be delayed until at least 15 minutes after the gastrokinetic medication and until the headache has built up to a mild-to-moderate intensity. Premature treatment leads to too frequent use of analgesics or vasoconstrictors, which over time increases the frequency of the headaches. Delayed treatment leads to a high frequency of unsuccessful treatments due to the impaired absorption of the medications. The treatment of the headache should be first attempted with a simple analgesic (e.g., aspirin, acetaminophen, or ibuprofen). In the absence of contraindications (e.g., peptic ulcer disease or bleeding disorder), aspirin or ibuprofen should be used, as they are most effective. Aspirin can be used in a dose of 1,000 mg, followed twice if necessary by 500 mg with intervals of a half hour. Ibuprofen can be used in a dose of 400 mg, repeated twice if necessary, also with intervals of a half hour. If acetaminophen is used, it can be given in the same dose as aspirin, that is, 1,000 mg followed twice if necessary by 500 mg with intervals of a half hour.

In the United States, in place of the simple analgesics or when aspirin or ibuprofen are contraindicated, Midrin can be used for the abortive treatment. Midrin is a combination preparation containing a mild vasoconstrictor (isometheptene), a mild sedative (dichloralphenazone), and acetaminophen. It is a nonaddicting preparation and is generally well-tolerated, with minimal or no adverse effects. It is most effective when given in a dose of two capsules, followed if necessary by one capsule every half hour with a maximum of six. If the patient tolerates the preparation well, it can be given in a dose of two capsules every half hour with a maximum of six. Midrin is contraindicated in patients treated with a monoamine oxidase inhibitor.

More potent than the simple analgesics and Midrin are the nonsteroidal anti-inflammatory analgesics. However, they are associated also with more adverse effects, in particular gastrointestinal upset. The nonsteroidal anti-inflammatory analgesics are, like aspirin and ibuprofen, contraindicated in peptic ulcer disease and bleeding disorder. Naproxen sodium is a good medication to use, as it is absorbed relatively rapidly. It can be used in a dose of 550 mg, followed twice if necessary by 275 mg with intervals of a half hour. The advantage of indomethacin is that it is also available as a rectal suppository. With the use of a rectal suppository, the stomach is bypassed, and the absorption is secured. Indomethacin can be used in a dose of 100 mg, followed twice if necessary by 50 mg with intervals of a half hour. The indomethacin suppository can cause an urge to defecate, but five to ten minutes in the rectum is enough for the medication to get absorbed. Indomethacin can cause orthostatic hypotension with lightheadedness when getting up too rapidly.

The indomethacin suppository also can be used when the headache is present on awakening in the morning or when it wakes the patient at night. Under such circumstances, the use of oral medications should be avoided, as they are likely to be ineffective due to the impaired absorption. However, if the headache is more than moderate-to-severe in intensity, indomethacin may not be potent enough to relieve it. More potent than indomethacin are the serotoninergic vasoconstrictors ergotamine, dihydroergotamine, and sumatriptan. Ergotamine is available as a rectal suppository in combination with caffeine (Cafergot). Dihydroergotamine and sumatriptan are available for parenteral administration. The medications are contraindicated in patients with hypertension or coronary artery disease and in those with significant risk factors for cardiovascular disease, as they are potent arterial vasoconstrictors.

The choice of the serotoninergic vasoconstrictor depends on the duration of the headaches. If the duration of the headaches is relatively short (12 to 24 hours or less), sumatriptan is the medication of choice. It is administered by subcutaneous injection in a dose of 6 mg. It is available with an auto-injector for easy administration by the patients themselves at home. It has a rapid onset of action and generally provides relief within one hour. If necessary, the injection can be repeated after one hour, but this generally does *not* increase the efficacy of the medication. Sumatriptan is well-tolerated by most patients, though it often causes a rush through the body within minutes of administration. The rush concentrates on the upper part of the body (upper chest, anterior neck, and face), where it causes a sensation of warmth or tingling. There may also be a pressure, heaviness, or tightness in these areas, an effect probably caused by contraction of skeletal muscles. The adverse effects, however, generally last only five to ten minutes.

Sumatriptan is short-acting, has a half-life of two hours, and is eliminated from the plasma in ten hours. This short half-life is associated with a relatively short duration of action and headache recurrence when the natural duration of the headache is longer than 12 to 24 hours. Certainly, the medication can be repeated, and up to two injections can be given in 24 hours. However, a longer-acting medication also can be used, such as ergotamine or dihydroergotamine. These medications have a plasma half-life of two hours as well but cause vasoconstriction for at least three days. However, though they generally provide longer relief of the headache than sumatriptan, they are not as well-tolerated, and the onset of their effect is not as rapid.

Ergotamine and (to a lesser extent) dihydroergotamine are notorious for causing nausea and vomiting. Patients usually do not tolerate an entire Cafergot suppository and, therefore, they should take only one-third of a suppository at a time. The one-third of the suppository can be repeated if necessary every half to one hour with a maximum of two suppositories in 24 hours.

Dihydroergotamine can be given by intranasal spray or by subcutaneous, intramuscular, or intravenous injection. When patients administer the medication themselves at home, either the intranasal spray or subcutaneous injection is preferred. The medication is given in a dose of 1 mg, which can be repeated if necessary once after one hour. When using it in the office, it is best to administer the medication by intramuscular injection. I *always* pretreat the patient with an antiemetic such as metoclopramide, 10 mg intramuscularly or intravenously. After 15 minutes, I give the dihydroergotamine in a dose of 0.5 intramuscularly, which I repeat if necessary after a half hour. Intravenous administration of the medication is associated with more adverse effects, in particular nausea and vomiting, and, hence, with a lower efficacy.

The ergot medications can also be given *after* the sumatriptan when the headache does return. The minimum time interval between the administration of sumatriptan and that of an ergot medication is one hour. No purpose would be served in giving the sumatriptan *after* an ergot medication.

TABLE 4.10
Summary of abortive migraine treatment

Headache comes about during the day
  Domperidone 20 mg or metoclopramide 10 mg by mouth during the migraine aura or at the onset of the headache, followed by
  Aspirin or acetaminophen, 1,000 mg by mouth, followed, if necessary, twice by 500 mg with intervals of a half hour, or
  Ibuprofen, 400 mg by mouth, repeated, if necessary, twice with intervals of a half hour, or
  Isometheptene (Midrin), two capsules by mouth, followed, if necessary, by one capsule every half hour with a maximum of six capsules, or
  Naproxen sodium, 550 mg by mouth, followed, if necessary, twice by 275 mg with intervals of a half hour, or
  Indomethacin, 100 mg by rectum, followed, if necessary, twice by 50 mg with intervals of a half hour, or
  Sumatriptan, 25–100 mg by mouth, repeated, if necessary, with minimal intervals of one hour with a maximum of 300 mg in 24 hours

Headache is present on awakening or wakes the patient at night
  Indomethacin, 100 mg by rectum, followed, if necessary, twice by 50 mg with intervals of a half hour, or
  Sumatriptan, 6 mg by subcutaneous injection, repeated, if necessary, once with a minimal interval of one hour, or
  Ergotamine (Cafergot), one-third suppository by rectum, repeated, if necessary, with intervals of a half to one hour with a maximum of two suppositories in 24 hours, or
  Dihydroergotamine, 1 mg subcutaneously or 0.5 mg intramuscularly, repeated, if necessary, once with an interval of a half to one hour

This is also potentially dangerous because of the long duration of the vasoconstrictor effect of the ergot medications.

No purpose is served either in giving the sumatriptan by injection unless the headache is moderate or severe in intensity. Early treatment of the headache with sumatriptan can be done with the use of the tablet. The tablet contains 25, 50, or 100 mg sumatriptan and up to 100 mg can be taken with minimal intervals of one hour with a maximum of 300 mg in 24 hours. The sumatriptan tablet is less effective than the sumatriptan injection, and the effect takes from two to four hours, instead of one hour, to develop.

When given during the aura, sumatriptan does *not* prolong the duration of the aura and also does not affect it otherwise.[66] It also does *not* prevent the development of the headache following the aura when administered during it!

The suggested sequence of use of the abortive antimigraine medications and their dosages are summarized in Table 4.10. (The medications under B can also be used when those under A fail to provide adequate relief.) When the headache returns after use of the sumatriptan injection, the Cafergot suppository or dihydroergotamine injection can be used to prevent further recurrence. A minimal interval of one hour is required between the sumatriptan injection and that of either Cafergot or dihydroergotamine.

References

1. Dexter SL. Rebreathing aborts migraine attacks. Br Med J 1982; 284:312.
2. Waelkens J. Domperidone in the prevention of complete classical migraine. Br Med J 1982; 284:944.
3. Laska EM, Sunshine A, Mueller F, et al. Caffeine as an analgesic adjuvant. JAMA 1984; 251:1711–1718.
4. Tfelt-Hansen P, Olesen J. Effervescent metoclopramide and aspirin (Migravess) versus effervescent aspirin or placebo for migraine attacks: A double-blind study. Cephalalgia 1984; 4:107–111.
5. Boureau F, Joubert JM, Lasserre V, et al. Double-blind comparison of an acetaminophen 400 mg–codeine 25 mg combination versus aspirin 1000 mg and placebo in acute migraine attack. Cephalalgia 1994; 14:156–161.
6. Peters BH, Fraim CJ, Masel BE. Comparison of 650 mg aspirin and 1,000 mg acetaminophen with each other, and with placebo in moderately severe headache. Am J Med 1983; 74(6A):36–42.
7. Chabriat H, Joire JE, Danchot J et al. Combined oral lysine acetylsalicylate and metoclopramide in the acute treatment of migrane: A multicentre double-blind placebo-controlled study. Cephalalgia 1994; 14:291–300.
8. Havanka-Kanniainen H. Treatment of acute migraine attack: Ibuprofen and placebo compared. Headache 1989; 29:507–509.
9. Kloster R, Nestvold K, Vilming ST. A double-blind study of ibuprofen versus placebo in the treatment of acute migraine attacks. Cephalalgia 1992; 12:169–171.

10. Pearce I, Frank GJ, Pearce JMS. Ibuprofen compared with paracetamol in migraine. Practitioner 1983; 227:465–467.
11. MacGregor EA, Wilkinson M, Bancroft K. Domperidone plus paracetamol in the treatment of migraine. Cephalalgia 1993; 13:124–127.
12. Tfelt-Hansen P, Olesen J, Aebelholt-Krabbe A, et al. A double blind study of metoclopramide in the treatment of migraine attacks. J Neurol Neurosurg Psychiatry 1980; 43:369–371.
13. Massiou H, Serrurier D, Lasserre O, Bousser MG. Effectiveness of oral diclofenac in the acute treatment of common migraine attacks: A double-blind study versus placebo. Cephalalgia 1991; 11:59–63.
14. Dahlof C, Bjorkman R. Diclofenac-K (50 and 100 mg) and placebo in the acute treatment of migraine. Cephalalgia 1993; 13:117–123.
15. Nelemans F. Een technisch gelukt onderzoek met indometacine bij patienten lijdende aan migraine. Een dubbelblind onderzoek versus placebo. Huisarts Wetenschap 1971; 14:337–340.
16. Sicuteri F, Michelacci S, Anselmi B. Termination of migraine headache by a new anti-inflammatory vasoconstrictor agent. Clin Pharmacol Ther 1965; 6:336–344.
17. Buzzi MG, Sakas DE, Moskowitz MA. Indomethacin and acetylsalicylic acid block neurogenic plasma protein extravasation in rat dura mater. Eur J Pharmacol 1989; 165:251–258.
18. Johnson ES, Ratcliffe DM, Wilkinson M. Naproxen sodium in the treatment of migraine. Cephalalgia 1985; 5:5–10.
19. Treves TA, Streiffler M, Korczyn AD. Naproxen sodium versus ergotamine tartrate in the treatment of acute migraine attacks. Headache 1992; 32:280–282.
20. Sargent JD, Baumel B, Peters K, et al. Aborting a migraine attack: Naproxen sodium v ergotamine plus caffeine. Headache 1988; 28:263–266.
21. Pradalier A, Rancurel G, Dordain G, et al. Acute migraine attack therapy: Comparison of naproxen sodium and an ergotamine tartrate compound. Cephalalgia 1985; 5:107–113.
22. Tokola RA, Kangasniemi P, Neuvonen PJ, Tokola O. Tolfenamic acid, metoclopramide, caffeine and their combinations in the treatment of migraine attacks. Cephalalgia 1984; 4:253–263.
23. Hakkarainen H, Vapaatalo H, Gothoni G, Parantainen J. Tolfenamic acid is as effective as ergotamine during migraine attacks. Lancet 1979; 2:326–328.
24. Diamond S, Freitag FG, Diamond ML, Urban G. Transnasal butorphanol in the treatment of migraine headache pain. Headache Q 1992; 3:164–171.
25. Hoffert MJ, Couch JR, Diamond S, et al. Transnasal butorphanol in the treatment of acute migraine. Headache 1995; 35:65–69.
26. Diamond S, Medina JL. Isometheptene—A non-ergot drug in the treatment of migraine. Headache 1975; 15:211–213.
27. Diamond S. Treatment of migraine with isometheptene, acetaminophen, and dichloralphenazone combination: a double-blind, crossover trial. Headache 1976; 15:282–287.
28. Yuill GM, Swinburn WR, Liversedge LA. A double-blind crossover trial of isometheptene mucate compound and ergotamine in migraine. Br J Clin Pract 1972; 26:76–79.

29. Edvinsson L, Jansen I. Characterization of 5-HT receptors mediating contraction of human cerebral, meningeal and temporal arteries: Target for GR 43175 in acute treatment of migraine. Cephalalgia 1989; 9 (suppl 10):39–40.
30. Chapman LF, Ramos AO, Goodell H, et al. A humoral agent implicated in vascular headache of the migraine type. Arch Neurol 1960; 3:223–229.
31. Saito K, Markowitz S, Moskowitz MA. Ergot alkaloids block neurogenic extravasation in dura mater: Proposed action in vascular headaches. Ann Neurol 1988; 24:732–737.
32. Buzzi MG, Moskowitz MA. The antimigraine drug, sumatriptan (GR 43175), selectively blocks neurogenic plasma extravasation from blood vessels in dura mater. Br J Pharmacol 1990; 99:202–206.
33. Maier HW. L'ergotamine inhibiteur du sympathique étudié en clinique comme moyen d'exploration et comme agent thérapeutique. Rev Neurol 1926; 33:1104–1108.
34. Graham JR, Wolff HG. Mechanism of migraine headache and action of ergotamine tartrate. Arch Neurol Psychiatry 1938; 39:737–763.
35. Waters WE. Controlled clinical trial of ergotamine tartrate. Br Med J 1970; 2:325–327.
36. Schmidt R, Fanchamps A. Effect of caffeine on intestinal absorption of ergotamine in man. Eur J Clin Pharmacol 1974; 7:213–216.
37. Friedman AP, DiSerio FJ, Hwang DS. Symptomatic relief of migraine: Multicenter comparison of Cafergot P-B, Cafergot, and placebo. Clin Ther 1989; 11:170–182.
38. Blowers AJ, Cameron EGM, Lawrence ER. Effervescent ergotamine tartrate (Effergot) in the treatment of the acute migraine attack. Br J Clin Pract 1981; 35:188–190.
39. Graham JR. Rectal use of ergotamine tartrate and caffeine alkaloid for the relief of migraine. N Engl J Med 1954; 250:936–938.
40. Hakkarainen H, Allonen H. Ergotamine vs. metoclopramide vs. their combination in acute migraine attacks. Headache 1982; 22:10–12.
41. Speed WG. Ergotamine tartrate inhalation: A new approach to the management of recurrent vascular headaches. Am J Med Sci 1960; 240:327–331.
42. Meyers L, Craft GS. Effectiveness of aerosol administration of ergotamine tartrate in migraine headache. N Y State J Med 1962; 62:1291–1293.
43. Horton BT, Peters GA, Blumenthal LS. A new product in the treatment of migraine: A preliminary report. Proceedings of the Staff Meetings of the Mayo Clinic 1945; 20:241–248.
44. Boissier JR. General pharmacology of ergot alkaloids. Pharmacology 1978; 16 (suppl 1):12–26.
45. Tulunay FC, Karan O, Aydin N, et al. Dihydroergotamine nasal spray during migraine attacks. A double-blind crossover study with placebo. Cephalalgia 1987; 7:131–133.
46. Ziegler D, Ford R, Kriegler J, et al. Dihydroergotamine nasal spray for the acute treatment of migraine. Neurology 1994; 44:447–453.
47. Dihydroergotamine Nasal Spray Multicenter Investigators. Efficacy, safety, and tolerability of dihydroergotamine nasal spray as monotherapy in the treatment of acute migraine. Headache 1995; 35:177–184.

48. Callaham M, Raskin N. A controlled study of dihydroergotamine in the treatment of acute migraine headache. Headache 1986; 26:168–171.
49. Scherl ER, Wilson JF. Comparison of dihydroergotamine with metoclopramide versus meperidine with promethazine in the treatment of acute migraine. Headache 1995; 35:256–259.
50. Saadah HA. Abortive headache therapy with intramuscular dihydroergotamine. Headache 1992; 32:18–20.
51. Hartman MM. Parenteral use of dihydroergotamine in migraine. Ann Allergy 1945; 3:440–442.
52. Bell R, Montoya D, Shuaib A, Lee MA. A comparative trial of three agents in the treatment of acute migraine headache. Ann Emerg Med 1990; 19:1079–1082.
53. Belgrade MJ, Ling LJ, Schleevogt MB, et al. Comparison of single-dose meperidine, butorphanol, and dihydroergotamine in the treatment of vascular headache. Neurology 1989; 39:590–592.
54. Doenicke A, Brand J, Perrin VL. Possible benefit of GR 43175, a novel 5-HT$_1$-like receptor agonist, for the acute treatment of severe headache. Lancet 1988; 1:1309–1311.
55. Jansen I, Edvinsson L, Mortensen A, Olesen J. Sumatriptan is a potent vasoconstrictor of human dural arteries via a 5-HT$_1$-like receptor. Cephalalgia 1992; 12:202–205.
56. McCarthy BG, Peroutka SJ. Comparative neuropharmacology of dihydroergotamine and sumatriptan (GR 43175). Headache 1989; 29:420–422.
57. Oral Sumatriptan Dose-Defining Study Group. Sumatriptan—An oral dose-defining study. Eur Neurol 1991; 31:300–305.
58. Ferrari MD, James MH, Bates D, et al. Oral sumatriptan: Effect of a second dose, and incidence and treatment of headache recurrences. Cephalalgia 1994; 14:330–338.
59. Oral Sumatriptan and Aspirin plus Metoclopramide Comparative Study Group. A study to compare oral sumatriptan with oral aspirin plus metoclopramide in the acute treatment of migraine. Eur Neurol 1992; 32:177–184.
60. Multinational Oral Sumatriptan and Cafergot Comparative Study Group. A randomized, double-blind comparison of sumatriptan and Cafergot in the acute treatment of migraine. Eur Neurol 1991; 31:314–322.
61. Finnish Sumatriptan Group and Cardiovascular Clinical Research Group. A placebo-controlled study of intranasal sumatriptan for the acute treatment of migraine. Eur Neurol 1991; 31:332–338.
62. Cady RK, Wendt JK, Kirchner JR, et al. Treatment of acute migraine with subcutaneous sumatriptan. JAMA 1991; 265:2831–2835.
63. Subcutaneous Sumatriptan International Study Group. Treatment of migraine attacks with sumatriptan. N Engl J Med 1991; 325:316–321.
64. Sumatriptan Auto-Injector Study Group. Self-treatment of acute migraine with subcutaneous sumatriptan using an auto-injector device. Eur Neurol 1991; 31:323–331.
65. Russell MB, Holm-Thomsen OE, Rishoj Nielsen M, et al. A randomized double-blind placebo-controlled crossover study of subcutaneous sumatriptan in general practice. Cephalalagia 1994; 14:291–296.

66. Bates D, Ashford E, Dawson R, et al. Subcutaneous sumatriptan during the migraine aura. Neurology 1994; 44:1587–1592.
67. Kaufman J, Levine I. Acute gastric dilatation of the stomach during attack of migraine. Radiology 1936; 27:301–302.
68. Boyle R, Behan PO, Sutton JA. A correlation between severity of migraine and delayed gastric emptying measured by an epigastric impedance method. Br J Clin Pharmacol 1990; 30:405–409.
69. Volans GN. The effect of metoclopramide on the absorption of effervescent aspirin in migraine. Br J Clin Pharmacol 1975; 2:57–63.
70. Tokola RA. The effect of metoclopramide and prochlorperazine on the absorption of effervescent paracetamol in migraine. Cephalalgia 1988; 8:139–147.
71. Pini LA, Bertolotti M, Trenti T, Vitale G. Disposition of naproxen after oral administration during and between migraine attacks. Headache 1993; 33:191–194.
72. Tokola RA, Neuvonen PJ. Effects of migraine attack and metoclopramide on the absorption of tolfenamic acid. Br J Clin Pharmacol 1984; 17:67–75.
73. Volans GN. Absorption of effervescent aspirin during migraine. Br Med J 1974; 4:265–269.
74. Tfelt-Hansen P, Paalzow L. Intramuscular ergotamine: Plasma levels and dynamic activity. Clin Pharmacol Ther 1985; 37:29–35.
75. Mueller-Schweinitzer E, Weidmann H. Regional differences in the responsiveness of isolated arteries from cattle, dog and man. Agents Actions 1977; 7:383–389.
76. Tfelt-Hansen P, Aebelholt-Krabbe A. Ergotamine abuse. Do patients benefit from withdrawal? Cephalalgia 1981; 1:29–32.

CHAPTER 5

Preventive Pharmacological Treatment

Preventive treatment refers to treatment of the migraine attack pattern. It involves the daily intake of a medication for either a shorter (short-term prevention) or longer period of time (long-term prevention). Short-term prevention is used when attacks occur at predictable times, for example, during menstruation, on weekends, during stressful periods, etc. It employs medications that have a relatively fast onset of action, such as the ergot alkaloids or anti-inflammatory medications (*vide infra*).

Long-term preventive treatment generally is indicated when migraine attacks occur more often than twice per month. However, it also depends on the intensity and duration of the attacks and on the effectiveness with which the attacks can be treated abortively. Preventive treatment generally results in a decrease in frequency of the attacks and, to a lesser extent, in a decrease in the intensity and duration. However, with effective preventive treatment, often the attacks that break through also can be treated more effectively abortively.

Long-term preventive treatment generally has to be continued for at least six months, after which time the dose can be decreased very gradually. Sometimes it is possible to maintain the improvement with a lower dose of the medication, or the medication can be discontinued fully without relapse of the condition. The medications that are effective in the preventive treatment of migraine can be divided into seven groups: ergot alkaloids, serotonin antagonists, beta-receptor blockers, tricyclic antidepressant, anti-inflammatory medications, calcium-entry blockers, and miscellaneous medications (Table 5.1). The medications are reviewed here in an order that is, however, determined more by their historic significance than by their relative efficacy.

TABLE 5.1
Medications effective in the preventive treatment of migraine

Ergot alkaloids
  Ergotamine (not available in the UK; Bellergal, US)
  Dihydroergotamine (Dihydergot, UK; not available in the US)
  Methysergide (Deseril, UK; Sansert, US)
Serotonin antagonists
  Cyproheptadine (Periactin, UK/US)
  Pizotifen (Sanomigran, UK; not available in the US)
Beta-receptor blockers
  Atenolol (Tenormin, UK/US)
  Metoprolol (Betaloc, UK; Lopressor, UK/US)
  Nadolol (Corgard, UK/US)
  Propranolol (Inderal, UK/US)
  Timolol (Betim, UK; Blocadren, US)
Tricyclic antidepressants
  Amitriptyline (Tryptizol, UK; Elavil, US)
Anti-inflammatory medications
  Aspirin (acetylsalicylic acid)
  Fenoprofen (Progesic, UK; Nalfon, US)
  Naproxen sodium (Synflex, UK; Anaprox, US)
Calcium-entry blockers
  Flunarizine (Sibelium; not available in the UK or US)
  Nicardipine (Cardene, UK/US)
  Nifedipine (Adalat, UK/US; Procardia, US)
  Nimodipine (Nimotop, UK/US)
  Verapamil (Cordilox, UK; Isoptin, US)
Miscellaneous medications
  Clonidine (Catapres, UK/US)
  Valproate (Epilim, UK; Depakote, US)

Ergot Alkaloids

The ergot alkaloids that are effective in the preventive treatment of migraine are ergotamine, dihydroergotamine, and methysergide. A summary of the reported efficacies of methysergide is presented in Table 5.2.

Ergotamine

Ergotamine is available in the US for the preventive treatment of migraine in the combination preparation *Bellergal-S*, which contains 0.6 mg ergotamine, 40 mg phenobarbital, and 0.2 mg belladonna alkaloids. The preparation was studied in a double-blind, placebo-controlled, *crossover* and *parallel* trial.[1] The trial involved 76 patients, 55 of whom completed the

TABLE 5.2
Reported efficacies of methysergide in the preventive treatment of migraine

Dose	Efficacy	Study
3 mg/day	28 percent decrease in attack frequency from pretrial condition	Andersson, 1973[8]
6 mg/day	Number of headache days 48 percent lower than during placebo treatment	Shekelle & Ostfeld, 1964[4]
6 mg/day	Number of severe headaches 30 percent lower than during placebo treatment	Southwell et al., 1964[5]
6 mg/day	Number of attacks 25 percent lower than during placebo treatment	Pedersen & Moller, 1966[6]

study. The dose of the medication was one tablet two times per day. The treatment periods were two weeks in the crossover part and four weeks in the parallel part. In the crossover part, the preparation was more effective than placebo. However, this was not the case in the parallel part, which reflects the lower sensitivity of that study design. In comparison to placebo, Bellergal-S decreased the intensity of the headaches by eight percent and increased the number of days without headache medications by 21 percent. The overall efficacy was rated by the patients as 21 percent higher for Bellergal-S than for placebo.

In an *open* study of 174 patients, the preparation was given in a dose of one-half tablet three times per day for six months.[2] The efficacy of Bellergal-S was 34 percent in substantially improving the headaches or rendering the patients headache-free (Table 5.3).

Dihydroergotamine

Dihydroergotamine (Dihydergot, UK, not available in the US) was studied in a double-blind, placebo-controlled, *parallel* trial.[3] The trial involved 40 patients, all of whom completed the study. The dose of the medication was 5 mg two times per day. The treatment periods were 30 days in duration. In comparison to the pretrial condition, the number of attacks decreased by 61 percent during treatment with dihydroergotamine and by 9 percent during placebo treatment. The intensity of the attacks was 67 percent lower during treatment with dihydroergotamine than during placebo treatment. The overall efficacy of the treatment was rated as sufficient by 65 percent of the patients in the dihydroergotamine group and by 10 percent in the placebo group.

TABLE 5.3
Effects on migraine prevention (open trial) of six months of treatment with placebo, Bellergal-S, methysergide, or cyproheptadine

	Placebo	Bellergal-S	Methysergide	Cyproheptadine
Free of headache	2 percent	10 percent	26 percent	16 percent
Substantially improved	18 percent	24 percent	29 percent	34 percent
No change	80 percent	66 percent	45 percent	50 percent
Number of patients	50	174	137	92

From Curran and Lance, 1964 with permission.[2]

Methysergide

Methysergide (Deseril, UK; Sansert, US) was studied in three double-blind, placebo-controlled, *crossover* trials. The first trial involved 18 patients, 13 of whom completed the study.[4] The dose of the medication was 2 mg three times per day. The treatment periods were five weeks in duration. The number of days with headache was 48 percent lower during treatment with methysergide than during placebo treatment.

The second trial involved 53 patients, 34 of whom completed the study.[5] The dose of the medication was 6 mg per day. The treatment periods were six weeks in duration. The number of headaches was 14 percent lower during treatment with methysergide than during placebo treatment. The number of severe headaches was 30 percent lower during treatment with methysergide than during placebo treatment. Adverse effects of the medication were lightheadedness, nausea, and aching of the leg muscles.

The third trial involved 102 patients, 60 of whom completed the study.[6] The dose of the medication was 3 mg two times per day. The treatment periods were six weeks in duration. The number of attacks was 25 percent lower during treatment with methysergide than during placebo treatment. In addition, in comparison to the pretrial condition, 57 percent of the patients showed a decrease in attack frequency of at least 50 percent during treatment with methysergide and 27 percent during placebo treatment. Adverse effects of the medication were leg symptoms, fatigue, and cardiac symptoms.

Serotonin Antagonists

Cyproheptadine and pizotifen are the serotonin antagonists that are effective in the preventive treatment of migraine. A summary of the reported efficacies of pizotifen is presented in Table 5.4.

TABLE 5.4
Reported efficacies of pizotifen in the preventive treatment of migraine

Dose	Efficacy	Study
1.5 mg/day	39 percent decrease in attack frequency from pretrial condition	Andersson, 1973[8]
1.5 mg/day	33 percent decrease in attack frequency from *placebo* baseline	Vilming et al., 1985[20]
1.5 mg/day	29 percent decrease in attack frequency from *placebo* baseline	Havanka-Kanniainen et al., 1987[56]
1.5 mg/day	36 percent decrease in attack frequency from *placebo* baseline	Bellavance & Meloche, 1990[41]
2–3 mg/day	38 percent decrease in attack frequency from pretrial condition	Spierings & Messinger, 1988[47]
3 mg/day	58 percent decrease in the number of severe headaches from *placebo* baseline	Arthur & Hornabrook, 1971[7]

Cyproheptadine

Cyproheptadine (Periactin, UK/US) was studied only in an *open* trial that involved 100 patients, 92 of whom completed the study.[2] The dose of the medication ranged from 12 to 24 mg per day. The treatment period was six months in duration. The medication rendered 16 percent of the patients headache-free, and an additional 34 percent improved substantially, (i.e., the total response was 50 percent) (Table 5.2). The adverse effects of the medication were drowsiness, aching legs, swollen ankles, nausea, and weight gain.

Pizotifen

Pizotifen (Sanomigran, UK; not available in the US) was studied in ten double-blind, placebo-controlled, crossover, and parallel trials, the largest of which is reviewed here.[7] The trial used a *crossover* design and involved 63 patients, 52 of whom completed the study. The dose of the medication was 3 mg per day. The treatment periods were four weeks in duration, preceded by a baseline period of four weeks. The number of headaches decreased by 22 percent from baseline during treatment with pizotifen but increased by 8 percent during placebo treatment. The number of *severe* headaches decreased by 58 percent from baseline during treatment with pizotifen and by 28 percent during placebo treatment. Forty percent of the patients experienced a reduction in headache frequency of 50 percent or more from baseline during treatment with pizotifen and 12 percent during placebo treatment. Adverse effects were experienced by 42 percent of the patients during treatment with pizotifen and by 13 percent during placebo treatment. The most common adverse effects were drowsiness and depression. In addition, an increase in weight was experienced by 59 percent of the patients during treatment with pizotifen and by 33 percent during placebo treatment.

Pizotifen was compared with methysergide in four double-blind, *crossover* studies, the largest of which is reviewed here.[8] This trial involved 73 patients, 49 of whom completed the study. The dose of pizotifen was 0.5 mg three times per day; the methysergide dose was 1 mg three times per day. The treatment periods were three months in duration. In comparison to the pretrial condition, the reduction in attack frequency was 39 percent during treatment with pizotifen and 28 percent during treatment with methysergide. A reduction in attack frequency of more than 50 percent was experienced by 37 percent of the patients during treatment with pizotifen and by 31 percent during treatment with methysergide.

Beta-Receptor Blockers

The beta-receptor blockers that are effective in the preventive treatment of migraine are atenolol, metoprolol, nadolol, propranolol, and timolol. Summaries of the reported efficacies of the beta-blockers are presented in Tables 5.5–5.8.

Propranolol

Propranolol (Inderal, UK/US) was the first beta-blocker to be used in the preventive treatment of migraine. It was studied in several double-blind, placebo-controlled trials, two of which, both *crossover* trials, are reviewed here. The first trial involved 83 patients, 62 of whom completed the study.[9] The dose of the medication was 80 mg per day, increased if necessary to 160 mg per day. The treatment periods were four weeks in duration. With regard to overall efficacy, 55 percent of the patients preferred propranolol over placebo, and 27 percent preferred placebo over propranolol.

The second trial involved 67 patients, 41 of whom completed the study.[10] The dose of the medication ranged from 60 to 320 mg per day. The dose was established during a dose-finding period of six weeks, preceded by a baseline period of four weeks. The treatment periods were 12 weeks in duration. After the dose-finding period, which was completed by 62 patients, the migraine condition was improved by 42 percent from baseline (Figure 5.1). In the first sequence (propranolol followed by placebo), the condition was 47 percent better during treatment with propranolol than during placebo treatment. In the second sequence (placebo followed by propranolol), the condi-

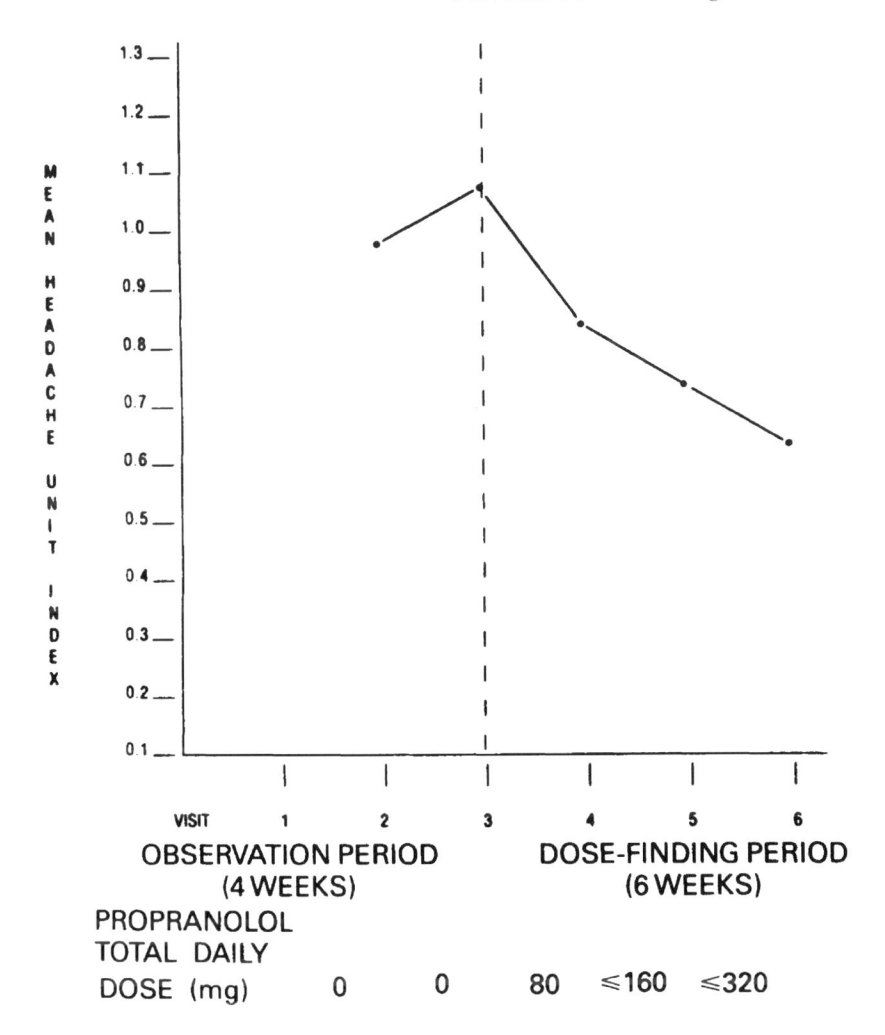

FIGURE 5.1 Mean headache unit index by visit before and during treatment with propranolol, 60 to 320 mg per day, in 62 patients with migraine. From Nadelmann JW, Stevens J, Saper JR. Propranolol in the prophylaxis of migraine. Headache 1986; 26:175-182 with permission.

tion was only 14 percent better during treatment with propranolol than during placebo treatment. With regard to adverse effects, 41 percent of the patients experienced fatigue during treatment with propranolol, 27 percent lethargy, 17 percent stomach upset, 16 percent nausea, 14 percent malaise, 11 percent diarrhea, 11 percent vivid dreams, 8 percent depressed mood, and 8 percent bradycardia.

Propranolol was studied in two double-blind, *crossover* trials in which a dose of 80 mg per day was compared with 160 mg per day. A long-acting

TABLE 5.5
Reported efficacies of propranolol in the preventive treatment of migraine

Dose	Efficacy	Study
80 mg/day	22 percent decrease in attack frequency from *placebo* baseline	Olsson et al., 1984[18]
80 mg/day	39 percent decrease in attack frequency from *placebo* baseline	Carroll et al., 1990[12]
120 mg/day	62–64 percent decrease in headache frequency from pretrial condition	Albers et al., 1989[53]
120 mg/day	39 percent decrease in number of attacks from *placebo* baseline	Ludin, 1989[48]
160 mg/day	Number of headache days 34 percent lower than during *placebo* treatment	Stensrud & Sjaastad, 1980[16]
160 mg/day	43 percent decrease in attack frequency from *placebo* baseline	Kangasniemi & Hedman, 1984[19]
160 mg/day	39 percent decrease in attack frequency from *placebo* baseline	Ryan, 1984[23]
160 mg/day	38 percent decrease in attack frequency from *placebo* baseline	Tfelt-Hansen et al., 1984[25]
160 mg/day	44 percent decrease in attack frequency from *placebo* baseline	Carroll et al., 1990[12]

preparation of the medication was administered once daily. The treatment periods were 12 weeks in duration, preceded by a *placebo* baseline period of four weeks. The first trial involved 48 patients, 42 of whom completed the study.[11] In comparison to the baseline period, 86 percent of the patients who took the 80 mg dose first and 81 percent of those who took the 160 mg dose first, experienced more than a 50 percent reduction in attack frequency during the first treatment period. Adverse effects of the medication were cold hands and feet, fatigue, and vivid dreams.

The second trial involved 51 patients, 37 of whom completed the study.[12] In comparison to the baseline period, the frequency of the attacks decreased by 39 percent during treatment with 80 mg propranolol and by 44 percent during treatment with 160 mg. The intensity and duration of the attacks was not affected by the medication in either dose. Adverse effects were

TABLE 5.6
Reported efficacies of metoprolol in the preventive treatment of migraine

Dose	Efficacy	Study
100 mg/day	22 percent decrease in attack frequency from *placebo* baseline	Olsson et al., 1984[18]
100 mg/day	31 percent decrease in attack frequency from *placebo* baseline	Louis et al., 1985[63]
100 mg/day	18 percent decrease in attack frequency from *placebo* baseline	Vilming et al., 1985[20]
200 mg/day	29 percent decrease in attack frequency from baseline	Andersson et al., 1983[17]
200 mg/day	43 percent decrease in attack frequency from *placebo* baseline	Kangasniemi & Hedman, 1984[19]
200 mg/day	50 percent decrease in the number of attacks from placebo baseline	Grotemeyer et al., 1990[37]
200 mg/day	37 percent decrease in the number of migraine days from *placebo* baseline	Soelberg Sorensen, et al., 1991[49]

experienced by 46 percent of the patients during treatment with 80 mg and by 65 percent during treatment with 160 mg. The most common adverse effect was fatigue.

Propranolol was compared with methysergide in a double-blind, *crossover* study.[13] The trial involved 56 patients, 36 of whom completed the study. The dose of propranolol was 40 mg three times per day; the dose of methysergide was 1 mg three times per day. The treatment periods were three months in duration. In comparison to the pretrial condition, 58 percent of the patients experienced a reduction in headache frequency of 50 percent or more during treatment with propranolol and 42 percent during treatment with methysergide. Adverse effects were experienced by 28 percent of the patients during treatment with propranolol and by 44 percent during treatment with methysergide.

Atenolol

Atenolol (Tenormin, UK/US) was studied in two double-blind, placebo-controlled, *crossover* trials. The dose of the medication was 100 mg once daily. The first trial involved 84 patients, 63 of whom completed the study.[14] The

TABLE 5.7
Reported efficacies of nadolol in the preventive treatment of migraine

Dose	Efficacy	Study
80 mg/day	41 percent decrease in attack frequency from *placebo* baseline	Ryan et al., 1983[21]
80 mg/day	55 percent decrease in attack frequency from *placebo* baseline	Ryan, 1984[23]
160 mg/day	45 percent decrease in attack frequency from *placebo* baseline	Ryan et al., 1983[21]
160 mg/day	47 percent decrease in attack frequency from *placebo* baseline	Ryan, 1984[23]
240 mg/day	61 percent decrease in attack frequency from *placebo* baseline	Ryan et al., 1983[21]

treatment periods were 12 weeks in duration. In comparison to placebo treatment, 33 percent of the patients experienced an improvement of more than 50 percent in their migraine condition during treatment with atenolol. No adverse effects occurred with the medication.

The second trial involved 24 patients, 20 of whom completed the study.[15] The treatment periods were three months in duration. In comparison to placebo treatment, 55 percent of the patients experienced an improvement of more than 50 percent in their migraine condition during treatment with atenolol. The number of attacks was 26 percent lower during treatment with atenolol than during placebo treatment. With regard to adverse effects, 30 percent of the patients experienced lightheadedness and 10 percent felt fatigue.

Atenolol was compared with propranolol in a double-blind, placebo-controlled, *crossover* trial.[16] The trial involved 35 patients, 28 of whom completed the study. The dose of atenolol was 50 mg two times per day; the propranolol dose was 80 mg two times per day. The treatment periods were six weeks in duration. In comparison to placebo treatment, the number of headache days was 14 percent lower during treatment with atenolol and 10 percent lower during treatment with propranolol. When the seven patients who experienced more than 15 days with headache during the six-week treatment periods were excluded, the number of headache days was 35 percent lower during treatment with atenolol and 34 percent lower during treatment with propranolol. Adverse effects were experienced by 4 percent of the patients during treatment with atenolol and by 43 percent during treatment with propranolol.

TABLE 5.8
Reported efficacies of atenolol and timolol in the preventive treatment of migraine

Medication	Efficacy	Study
Atenolol		
100 mg/day	Number of headache days 35 percent lower than during placebo treatment	Stensrud & Sjaastad, 1980[16]
100 mg/day	Number of attacks 26 percent lower than during placebo treatment	Forssman et al., 1983[15]
Timolol		
20 mg/day	44 percent decrease in attack frequency from baseline	Tfelt-Hansen et al., 1984[25]
20 mg/day	32 percent decrease in headache frequency from placebo baseline	Stellar et al., 1984[24]

Metoprolol

Metoprolol (Betaloc, UK; Lopressor, UK/US) was studied in a double-blind, placebo-controlled, *parallel* trial.[17] The trial involved 71 patients, 62 of whom completed the study. The dose of the medication was 200 mg (controlled-release preparation) once daily. The treatment periods were eight weeks in duration, preceded by a baseline period of four weeks. The frequency of the attacks decreased by 29 percent from baseline in the metoprolol group and by 10 percent in the placebo group. The number of days with migraine also decreased by 29 percent from baseline in the metoprolol group and by 2 percent in the placebo group. The overall efficacy of the treatment was rated as moderate or marked by 54 percent of the patients in the metoprolol group and by 18 percent in the placebo group. With regard to adverse effects, sleep disturbances, such as insomnia and nightmares, and fatigue were more frequently experienced by the patients in the metoprolol group than in the placebo group.

Metoprolol was compared with propranolol in two double-blind, *crossover* trials. The first trial involved 56 patients, 53 of whom completed the study.[18] The dose of metoprolol was 50 mg two times per day; the propranolol dose was 40 mg two times per day. The treatment periods were eight weeks in duration, preceded by a *placebo* baseline period of four weeks. The frequency of the attacks decreased by 22 percent from baseline during treatment with metoprolol and by 22 percent during treatment with propranolol. The number of days with migraine decreased by 25 percent from baseline during treatment with metoprolol and by 33 percent during treatment with propranolol. Adverse effects were experienced by 58 percent of the patients during treatment with metoprolol and by 58 percent during treatment with propranolol.

The second trial involved 36 patients, 33 of whom completed the study.[19] The dose of metoprolol was 200 mg once daily (controlled-release preparation); the propranolol dose was 80 mg two times per day. The treatment periods were eight weeks in duration, preceded by a *placebo* baseline period of four weeks. The frequency of the attacks decreased by 43 percent from baseline during treatment with metoprolol and by 43 percent during treatment with propranolol (Figure 5.2). The number of days with headache decreased by 46 percent from baseline during treatment with metoprolol and by 44 percent during treatment with propranolol. Adverse effects were experienced by 50 percent of the patients during treatment with metoprolol and by 56 percent during treatment with propranolol.

Metoprolol was compared with pizotifen in a double-blind, *crossover* study.[20] The trial involved 35 patients, 30 of whom completed the study. The dose of metoprolol was 50 mg two times per day; the dose of pizotifen was 0.5 mg three times per day. The treatment periods were eight weeks in duration, preceded by a *placebo* baseline period of four weeks. The frequency of the attacks decreased by 18 percent from baseline during treat-

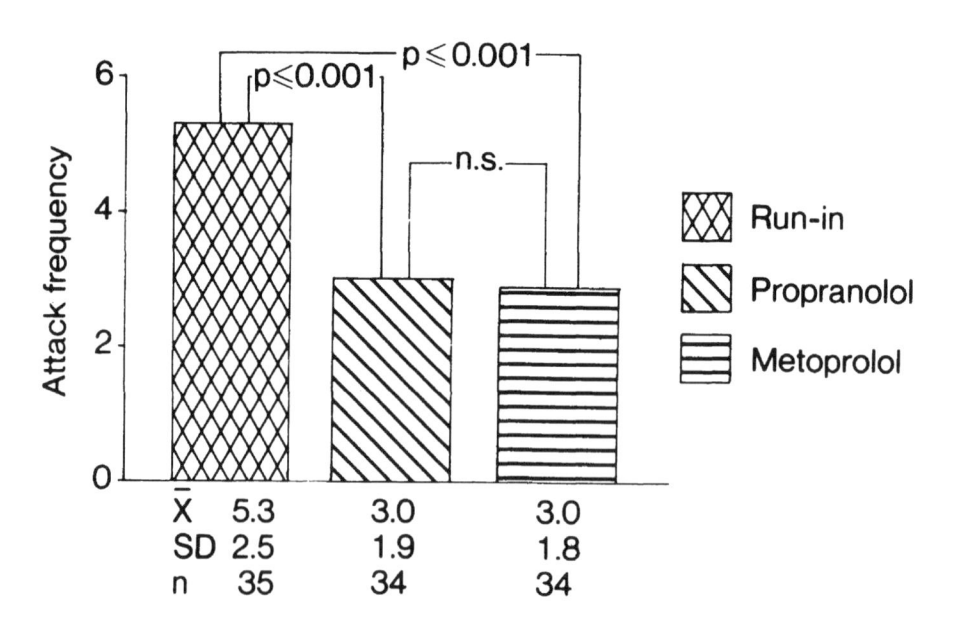

FIGURE 5.2 Frequency of migraine attacks during placebo baseline ("run-in") and during treatment with propranolol, 80 mg two times per day, and metoprolol, 200 mg once daily (controlled-release preparation). From Kangasniemi P, Hedman C. Metoprolol and propranolol in the prophylactic treatment of classical and common migraine. A double-blind study. Cephalalgia 1984; 4:91–96 with permission.

ment with metoprolol and by 33 percent during treatment with pizotifen (Figure 5.3). During treatment with metoprolol, 29 percent of the patients experienced an improvement of at least 50 percent in their migraine condition and 42 percent during treatment with pizotifen. Adverse effects were experienced by 44 percent of the patients during treatment with metoprolol and by 61 percent during treatment with pizotifen. During treatment with pizotifen, 50 percent of the patients experienced an increase in weight of more than two kilogram, as compared to 6 percent during treatment with metoprolol.

Nadolol

Nadolol (Corgard, UK/US) was studied in a double-blind, placebo-controlled, *parallel* trial.[21] The trial involved 80 patients, 79 of whom completed the study. The dose of the medication was 80, 160, or 240 mg per day. The treatment periods were three months in duration, preceded by a *placebo* baseline period of two months. The frequency of the attacks decreased by 39 percent from baseline in the placebo group and by 41 percent, 45 percent, and 61 percent, respectively, in the 80-, 160-, and 240-mg nadolol groups. Adverse ef-

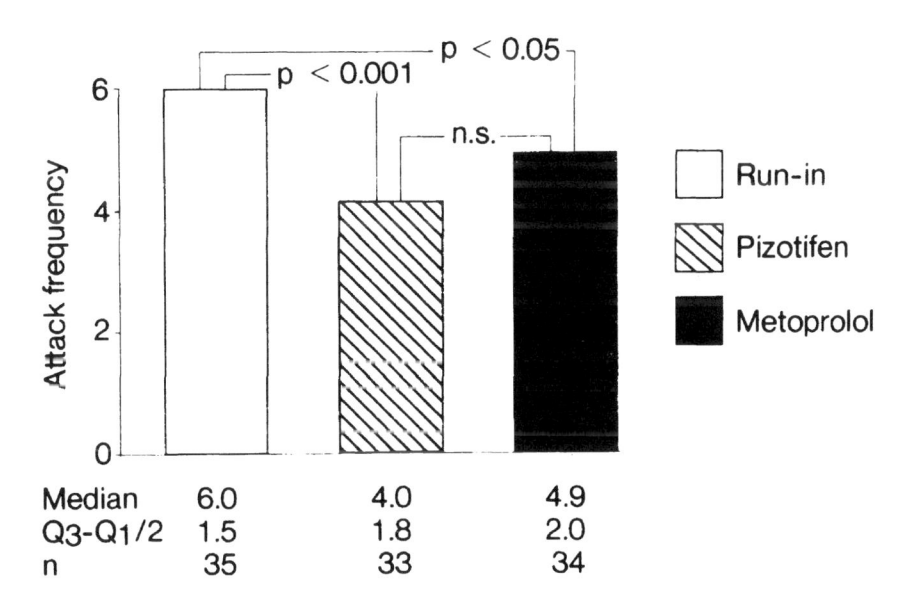

FIGURE 5.3 Frequency of migraine attacks during placebo baseline ("run-in") and during treatment with pizotifen, 0.5 mg three times per day, and metoprolol, 50 mg two times per day. From Vilming S, Standnes B, Hedman C. Metoprolol and pizotifen in the prophylactic treatment of classical and common migraine. A double-blind investigation. Cephalalgia 1985; 5:17–23 with permission.

fects were experienced by 25 percent of the patients in the placebo, 80-mg, and 160-mg nadolol groups and by 50 percent in the 240-mg group.

Nadolol was compared with propranolol in three double-blind, *parallel* studies, two of which are reviewed here. The first trial involved 140 patients, 98 of whom completed the study.[22] The dose of nadolol was 80 or 160 mg once daily; the propranolol dose was 80 mg two times per day. The treatment periods were 12 weeks in duration, preceded by a *placebo* baseline period of four to eight weeks. Thirty-six percent of the patients in the 80-mg nadolol group experienced a reduction in headache frequency of at least 50 percent from baseline, 52 percent of those in the 160-mg group, and 16 percent of those in the propranolol group. A reduction in headache intensity of at least 50 percent was experienced by 37 and 60 percent, respectively, of the patients in the 80-and 160-mg nadolol groups and by 32 percent of those in the propranolol group.

The second trial involved 48 patients, 45 of whom completed the study.[23] The dose of nadolol was 80 or 160 mg per day, the dose of propranolol was 160 mg per day. The treatment periods were 12 weeks in duration, preceded by a *placebo* baseline period of four weeks. The frequency of the headaches decreased by 55 percent from baseline in the 80-mg nadolol group, by 47 percent in the 160-mg group, and by 39 percent in the propranolol group.

Timolol

Timolol (Betim, UK; Blocadren, US) was studied in a double-blind, placebo-controlled, *crossover* trial.[24] The trial involved 107 patients, 94 of whom completed the study. The dose of the medication was 10 mg two times per day. The treatment periods were eight weeks in duration, preceded by a *placebo* baseline period of four weeks. The frequency of the headaches decreased by 32 percent from baseline during treatment with timolol and by 23 percent during placebo treatment. Forty-three percent of the patients experienced a reduction in headache frequency of at least 50 percent during treatment with timolol and 27 percent during placebo treatment. With regard to adverse effects, insomnia and fatigue were more common during treatment with timolol than during placebo treatment.

Timolol was compared with propranolol in a double-blind, placebo-controlled, *crossover* study.[25] The trial involved 96 patients, 83 of whom completed the study. The dose of timolol was 10 mg two times per day; the propranolol dose was 80 mg two times per day. The treatment periods were 12 weeks in duration, preceded by a baseline period of four weeks. The frequency of the attacks decreased by 44 percent from baseline during treatment with timolol, by 38 percent during treatment with propranolol, and by 19 percent during placebo treatment. The intensity of the attacks decreased by 10, 6, and 0 percent, respectively, and the duration of the attacks decreased by 15, 16, and 9 percent, respectively. Fifty-five percent of the patients experienced a reduction in headache frequency of at least 50 percent during treatment with timolol, 60 percent during treatment with propranolol, and 30 percent during placebo treatment. Adverse effects were experienced by 46 percent of the patients during treatment with timolol, by 42 percent during treatment with propranolol, and by 28 percent during placebo treatment. The most common adverse effects were fatigue, lightheadedness, sleep disturbances, nausea, and depression.

Tricyclic Antidepressants

The only tricyclic antidepressant that has been shown to be effective in the preventive treatment of migraine is *amitriptyline* (Tryptizol, UK; Elavil, US). It was studied in two double-blind, placebo-controlled trials. The first was a *crossover* trial and involved 26 patients, 20 of whom completed the study.[26] The dose of the medication ranged from 10 to 60 mg per day. The dose was established during a dose-finding period of four weeks. The patients were maintained on the optimal dose for 23 weeks. The number of attacks was 42 percent lower during treatment with amitriptyline than during placebo treatment. The number of *severe* attacks was 44 percent lower during treatment with amitriptyline than during placebo treatment. The effect of amitriptyline on the number of attacks was independent of the intensity of the attacks. The number of attacks shorter than 24 hours was 46 percent lower during treatment with amitriptyline than during placebo treatment, but the number of attacks longer than 24 hours was only 15 percent lower. Adverse effects were experienced by 80 percent of the patients during treatment with amitriptyline and by 70 percent during placebo treatment. The most common adverse effects were drowsiness and dry mouth.

The second was a *parallel* trial and involved 162 patients, 100 of whom completed the study.[27] The treatment periods were four weeks in duration, preceded by a *placebo* baseline period of four weeks. The dose of the medication ranged from 50 to 100 mg per day. Fifty-five percent of the patients in the amitriptyline group experienced an improvement of at least 50 percent in their migraine condition, as compared to 34 percent in the placebo group. The correlation between the changes in migraine and depression during treatment with amitriptyline was low but statistically significant, and there was no correlation during placebo treatment. The most common adverse effects of the medication were dry mouth, bad taste, and drowsiness.

Amitriptyline was compared with propranolol in a double-blind, placebo-controlled, *crossover* study.[28] The trial involved 54 patients, 30 of whom completed the study. The dose of amitriptyline ranged from 50 to 150 mg per day; the propranolol dose ranged from 80 to 240 mg per day. The treatment periods were four weeks in duration, preceded by a *placebo* baseline period of four weeks. In comparison to placebo treatment, 33 percent of the patients experienced an improvement of 50 percent or more in their migraine condition during treatment with amitriptyline and 40 percent during treatment with propranolol.

80   *Management of Migraine*

Amitriptyline was also compared with propranolol in a single-blind, *crossover* study.[29] The trial involved 30 patients, all of whom completed the study. The dose of amitriptyline ranged from 25 to 150 mg per day; the propranolol dose ranged from 40 to 240 mg per day. The treatment periods were eight weeks in duration, preceded by a *placebo* baseline period of four to eight weeks. Sixteen of the patients responded to both medications, six only to propranolol and eight only to amitriptyline. In the patients who only responded to amitriptyline, the medication decreased the frequency of the migraine headaches by 51 percent, the intensity by 20 percent, and the duration by 36 percent. In the patients who only responded to propranolol, the medication decreased the frequency of the migraine headaches by 1 percent, the intensity by 18 percent, and the duration by 17 percent. A response to amitriptyline was associated with a high frequency and short duration of the headaches and a response to propranolol with a long duration of the headaches. The effectiveness of the medications did *not* depend on the blood levels or on the reduction in saliva secretion (amitriptyline) or pulse rate response on exercise (propranolol).

Amitriptyline was compared with *fluvoxamine* (Faverin, UK; Luvox, US), a selective serotonin re-uptake inhibitor, in a double-blind, *parallel* study.[30] The study involved 70 patients, 44 of whom completed the study. The dose of amitriptyline was 25 mg at bed time; the fluvoxamine dose was 50 mg at bed time. The treatment periods were 12 weeks in duration, preceded by a *placebo* baseline period of four weeks. The number of headaches decreased by 40 percent from baseline during treatment with amitriptyline and by 56 percent during treatment with fluvoxamine. Adverse effect during treatment with amitriptyline was drowsiness (23 percent); during treatment with fluvoxamine adverse effects were drowsiness, dry mouth, nausea, and general weakness (15 percent).

Another selective serotonin re-uptake inhibitor that was studied in the preventive treatment of migraine but found *not* to be effective is *fluoxetine* (Prozac; UK/US). It was studied in a double-blind, placebo-controlled, *parallel* trial that involved 58 patients.[31] The dose of the medication was 20 or 40 mg per day. The treatment periods were three months in duration, preceded by a *placebo* baseline period of one month.

Clomipramine (Anafranil, UK/US) was studied in two double-blind, placebo-controlled, *crossover* trials. The first trial involved 21 patients, 10 of whom completed the study.[32] The dose of the medication was 10 mg three times per day. The treatment periods were eight weeks in duration. In comparison to the pretrial condition, the number of attacks decreased by 50 percent during treatment with clomipramine and by 42 percent during placebo treatment.

The second trial involved 63 patients, 36 of whom completed the study.[33] The dose of the medication was up to 100 mg per day. The treatment periods were four weeks in duration, preceded by a baseline period of six weeks. The number of attacks decreased by more than 50 percent from baseline in 57 percent of the patients during treatment with clomipramine and in 70 percent during placebo treatment.

Anti-inflammatory Medications

The anti-inflammatory medications that are effective in the preventive treatment of migraine are aspirin, naproxen sodium, tolfenamic acid, and fenoprofen.

Aspirin

Aspirin (acetylsalicylic acid) was studied in a double-blind, placebo-controlled, *crossover* trial.[34] The trial involved 12 patients, all of whom completed the study. The dose of the medication was 650 mg two times per day. The treatment periods were three months in duration. The number of headaches was 60 percent lower during treatment with aspirin than during placebo treatment.

Aspirin was also studied in a double-blind, placebo-controlled, *parallel* trial.[35] The trial was a population study of 22,071 male physicians who were treated with 325 mg aspirin every other day. Of the physicians in the aspirin group, 6 percent reported migraine attacks during the trial, compared to 7.4 percent in the placebo group, indicating a 20-percent difference.

Aspirin was compared with propranolol in a double-blind, *crossover* study.[36] The trial involved 18 patients, 12 of whom completed the study. The dose of aspirin was 13.5 mg/kg/day; the propranolol dose was 0.1 mg/kg/day. The treatment periods were three months in duration, preceded by a baseline period of one month. The migraine condition improved by 65 percent during treatment with aspirin and by 65 percent during treatment with propranolol.

Aspirin was compared with metoprolol in a double-blind, *crossover* study.[37] The trial involved 28 patients, 21 of whom completed the study. The dose of aspirin was 500 mg three times per day; the metoprolol dose was was 200 mg once daily. The treatment periods were 12 weeks in duration, preceded by a baseline period of eight weeks. The number of attacks decreased by 26 percent from baseline during treatment with aspirin and by 50 percent during treatment with metoprolol. Fourteen percent of the patients experienced a more than 50 percent reduction in attack frequency during treatment with aspirin and 67 percent during treatment with metoprolol.

Naproxen sodium

Naproxen sodium (Synflex, UK; Anaprox, US) was studied in two double-blind, placebo-controlled, *crossover* trials. The first trial involved 51 patients, 35 of whom completed the study.[38] The dose of the medication was 275 mg two times per day. The treatment periods were eight weeks in duration, preceded by a baseline period of two weeks. The number of days with headache was 16 percent lower during treatment with naproxen sodium than during placebo treatment, and the number of days with *severe* headache 50 percent. Adverse effects were experienced by 20 percent of the patients during treatment with naproxen sodium and by 20 percent during placebo treatment. The most common adverse effect of naproxen sodium was stomach upset.

The second trial involved 40 patients, 34 of whom completed the study.[39] The dose of the medication was 550 mg two times per day. The treatment periods were eight weeks in duration, preceded by a *placebo* baseline period of two weeks. With regard to overall efficacy, 50 percent of the patients rated naproxen sodium better than placebo, and 15 percent rated placebo better than naproxen sodium (Figure 5.4). Adverse effects were experienced by 14 percent of the patients during treatment with naproxen sodium and by 20 percent during placebo treatment.

Naproxen sodium was compared with propranolol in a double-blind, placebo-controlled, *parallel* study.[40] The trial involved 170 patients, 129 of

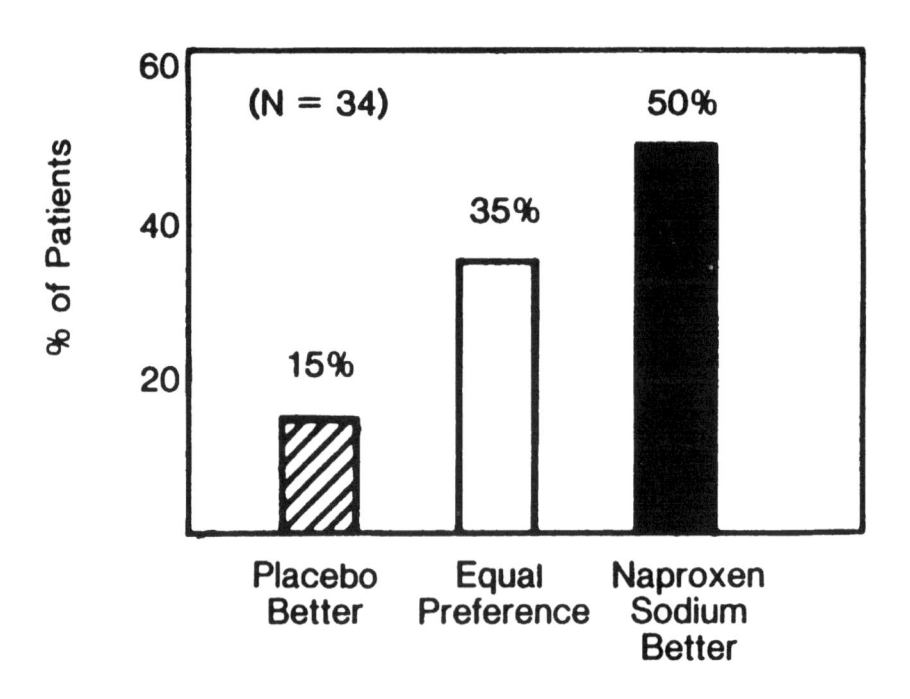

FIGURE 5.4 Patient preference of naproxen sodium, 550 mg two times per day, versus placebo in the preventive treatment of migraine. From Ziegler DK, Ellis DJ. Naproxen in prophylaxis of migraine. Arch Neurol 1985; 42:582–584 with permission.

whom completed the study. The dose of naproxen sodium was 550 mg two times per day; the propranolol dose was 40 mg three times per day. The treatment periods were 12 weeks in duration, preceded by a *placebo* baseline period of two weeks. Naproxen sodium and propranolol both showed trends toward superiority over placebo in reducing the number of days with headache as well as the intensity of the headaches. With regard to overall efficacy, the patients rated both medications superior to placebo. With regard to adverse effects, the patients in the naproxen-sodium group experienced more gastrointestinal upset than in the propranolol or placebo group.

Naproxen sodium was compared with pizotifen in a single-blind, placebo-controlled, *parallel* study.[41] The trial involved 318 patients, 176 of whom completed the study. The dose of naproxen sodium was 550 mg two times per day; the pizotifen dose was 0.5 mg three times per day. The treatment periods were 12 weeks in duration, preceded by a *placebo* baseline period of eight weeks. The frequency of the attacks decreased by 42 percent from baseline in the naproxen-sodium group, by 36 percent in the pizotifen group, and by 11 percent in the placebo group. The intensity of the attacks decreased by 19 percent from baseline in the naproxen-sodium group, by 9 percent in the pizotifen group, and by 6 percent in the placebo group. The duration of the attacks decreased by 19 percent from baseline in the naproxen-sodium group, by 5 percent in the pizotifen group, and by 2 percent in the placebo group. Adverse effects were experienced by 26 percent of the patients in the naproxen-sodium group, by 28 percent of those in the pizotifen group, and by 28 percent of those in the placebo group. The most common adverse effects were gastrointestinal upset in both the naproxen-sodium and pizotifen group, followed by weight gain in the pizotifen group.

Tolfenamic acid

Tolfenamic acid (not available in the UK or US) was studied in a double-blind, placebo-controlled, *crossover* trial.[42] The trial involved 38 patients, 31 of whom completed the study. The dose of the medication was 100 mg three times per day. The treatment periods were 10 weeks in duration, separated by an interval of two weeks. The frequency of the attacks was 27 percent lower during treatment with tolfenamic acid than during placebo treatment. The duration of the attacks was 23 percent shorter, and the median intensity was 21 percent lower. Gastrointestinal adverse effects occurred in 42 percent of the patients during treatment with tolfenamic acid and in 39 percent during placebo treatment.

Fenoprofen

Fenoprofen (Progesic, UK; Nalfon, US) was studied in a double-blind, placebo-controlled, *parallel* trial.[43] The trial involved 118 patients, 102 of whom completed the study. The dose of the medication was 200 or 600 mg three times per day. The treatment periods were 12 weeks in duration, preceded by a *placebo* baseline period of four weeks. The headache frequency decreased by at least 50 percent from baseline in 22 percent of the patients in the 200-mg group, in 36 percent of those in the 600-mg group, and in 20 percent of those in the placebo group. With regard to adverse effects, gastrointestinal symptoms, including abdominal pain, dyspepsia, and flatulence, were experienced by 10 percent of the patients in the 200-mg group, by 14 percent of those in the 600-mg group, and by 4 percent of those in the placebo group. Fatigue and drowsiness were experienced by 16 percent of the patients in the 200-mg group, by 4 percent of those in the 600-mg group, and by 3 percent of those in the placebo group.

Indomethacin

Indomethacin (Indocid, UK; Indocin, US) was studied in a double-blind, placebo-controlled, *parallel* trial.[44] The trial involved 38 patients, all of whom completed the study. The dose of the medication was 25 mg three times per day. The treatment periods were one month in duration. Thirty-seven percent of the patients in the indomethacin group experienced an improvement of at least 50 percent in their migraine condition, as compared to 37 percent of those in the placebo group. With regard to adverse effects, 37 percent of the patients in the indomethacin group experienced indigestion, 26 percent felt lightheaded, 26 percent reported insomnia, and 26 percent complained of fullness in the head. The last adverse effect was also experienced by 21 percent of the patients in the placebo group.

Calcium-Entry Blockers

The calcium-entry blockers that are effective in the preventive treatment of migraine are flunarizine, nicardipine, nifedipine, nimodipine, and verapamil. A summary of the reported efficacies of flunarizine is presented in Table 5.9.

Flunarizine

Flunarizine (Sibelium; not available in the UK or US) was studied in several double-blind, placebo-controlled trials, the largest two of which are reviewed here. The first was a *parallel* trial and involved 58 patients, all of whom completed the study.[45] The dose of the medication was 5 mg two times per day. The treatment periods were three months in duration. In comparison to the pretrial condition, the frequency of the attacks decreased by 57 percent in the flunarizine group and by 14 percent in the placebo group. The number of days with *severe* headache also decreased more prominently in the flunarizine group than in the placebo group (Figure 5.5). Ad-

TABLE 5.9
Reported efficacies of flunarizine in the preventive treatment of migraine

Dose	Efficacy	Study
10 mg/day	57 percent decrease in attack frequency from pretrial condition	Louis, 1981[45]
10 mg/day	43 percent decrease in attack frequency from baseline	Soelberg Sorensen, et al., 1986[46]
10 mg/day	46 percent decrease in attack frequency from pretrial condition	Spierings & Messinger, 1988[47]
10 mg/day	27 percent decrease in the number of attacks from *placebo* baseline	Ludin, 1989[48]
10 mg/day	37 percent decrease in the number of migraine days from *placebo* baseline	Soelberg Sorensen, et al., 1991[49]

verse effects were experienced by 7 percent of the patients in each group and consisted of mild drowsiness in the flunarizine group.

The second was a *crossover* trial and included 29 patients, 27 of whom completed the study.[46] The dose of the medication was 10 mg once daily. The treatment periods were 16 weeks in duration, preceded by a baseline period of four weeks. The frequency of the attacks decreased by 43 percent from baseline during treatment with flunarizine and by 9 percent during placebo treatment. The intensity and duration of the attacks were not affected by the treatments. Adverse effects were experienced by 11 percent of the patients during treatment with flunarizine and by 4 percent during placebo treatment. The adverse effect consisted of mild daytime drowsiness.

Flunarizine was compared with pizotifen in six double-blind, parallel or crossover studies. Three of these trials employed the same protocol and were combined in a secondary analysis of the results.[47] They were *parallel* trials and involved 74 patients in the flunarizine group and 60 in the pizotifen group. The dose of flunarizine was 10 mg per day; the pizotifen dose was 2 to 3 mg per day. The treatment periods were three or four months in duration. In comparison to the pretrial condition, the frequency of the attacks decreased by 46 percent in the flunarizine group and by 38 percent in the pizotifen group.

Flunarizine was compared with propranolol in a double-blind, *parallel* study.[48] The trial involved 71 patients, 59 of whom completed the study. The dose of flunarizine was 10 mg once daily; the propranolol dose was 40 mg three times per day. The treatment periods were four months in duration, preceded by a *placebo* baseline period of one month. Considering the

86 *Management of Migraine*

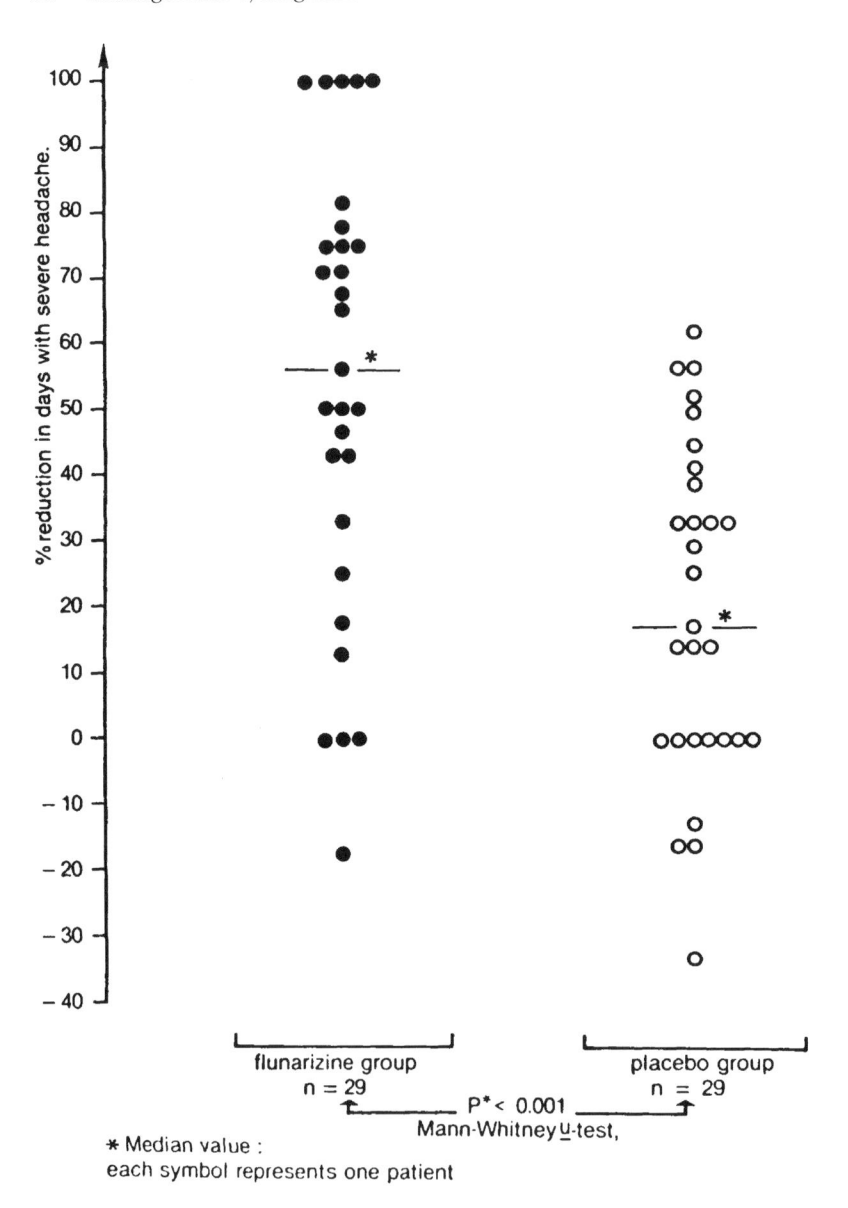

FIGURE 5.5 Percentage reduction in days with severe headache from pretrial condition during treatment with flunarizine, 5 mg two times per day, as compared to placebo. From Louis P. A double-blind placebo-controlled prophylactic study of flunarizine (Sibelium) in migraine. Headache 1981; 21:235–239 with permission.

last month of treatment only, the number of attacks decreased by 27 percent from baseline in the flunarizine group and by 39 percent in the propranolol group. The intensity of the attacks decreased by 12 and 25 percent from baseline, respectively, while the duration of the attacks increased by 27 percent in the flunarizine group and decreased by 23 percent in the propranolol group. Adverse effects were experienced by 48 percent of the patients in the flunarizine group and by 47 percent of those in the propranolol group. The most common adverse effect in the flunarizine group was drowsiness, and in the propranolol group it was gastrointestinal upset.

Flunarizine was compared with metoprolol in a double-blind, *parallel* study.[49] The trial involved 149 patients, 127 of whom completed the study. The dose of flunarizine was 10 mg once daily; the metoprolol dose was 200 mg once daily. The treatment periods were 16 weeks in duration, preceded by a *placebo* baseline period of four weeks. The number of days with migraine decreased by 37 percent from baseline in the flunarizine group and by 37 percent in the metoprolol group. The intensity of the attacks decreased by 16 and 19 percent from baseline, respectively, and the duration decreased by 23 and 29 percent, respectively. With regard to adverse effects, drowsiness was experienced by 36 percent of the patients in the flunarizine group and by 28 percent of those in the metoprolol group. Weight gain was experienced by 32 percent of the patients in the flunarizine group and by 12 percent of those in the metoprolol group. Depression was the most serious adverse effect and was experienced by 8 percent of the patients in the flunarizine group and by 3 percent of those in the metoprolol group.

Nicardipine

Nicardipine (Cardene, UK/US) was studied in a double-blind, placebo-controlled, *crossover* trial.[50] The trial involved 30 patients, 24 of whom completed the study. The dose of the medication was 20 mg two times per day. The treatment periods were two months in duration, preceded by a baseline period of two months. The frequency of the attacks decreased by 62 percent from baseline during treatment with nicardipine and by 23 percent during treatment with placebo. The intensity of the attacks decreased by 50 and 0 percent from baseline, respectively, and the duration by 72 and 36 percent, respectively. Adverse effects were equally common during treatment with nicardipine and during placebo treatment. The adverse effects were mostly lightheadedness and stomach upset.

Nifedipine

Nifedipine (Adalat, UK/US; Procardia, US) was studied in a double-blind, placebo-controlled, *crossover* trial.[51] The trial involved only eight patients, all of whom completed the study. The dose of the medication was 10 mg three times per day. The treatment periods were one month in duration, preceded by a baseline period of one month. The frequency of the attacks decreased by 75 percent from baseline during treatment with nifedipine and by

5 percent during placebo treatment (Figure 5.6). The intensity of the attacks decreased by 73 and 6 percent from baseline, respectively.

Nifedipine was compared with flunarizine in a double-blind, *parallel* study.[52] The trial involved 90 patients, 78 of whom completed the study. The dose of nifedipine was 10 mg two times per day; the flunarizine dose was 5 mg two times per day. The treatment periods were three months in duration, preceded by a *placebo* baseline period of one month. The migraine condition improved by 38 percent from baseline in the nifedipine group and

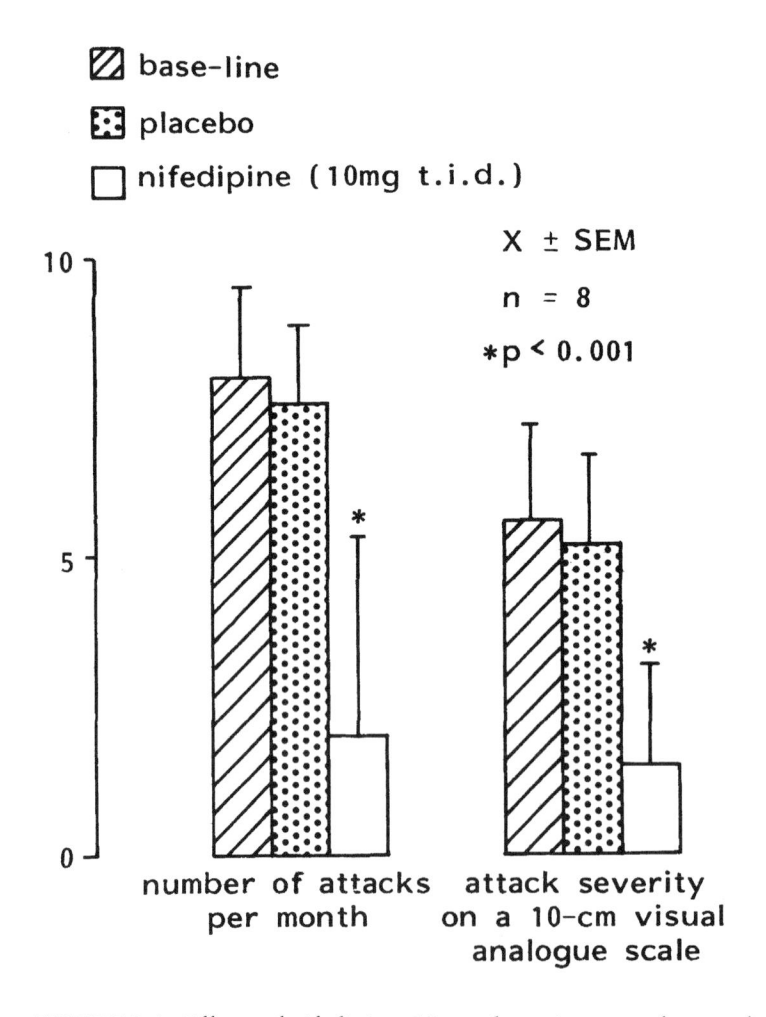

FIGURE 5.6 Effects of nifedipine, 10 mg three times per day, on the frequency (left) and intensity (right) of migraine attacks as compared with baseline and placebo treatment. Adapted from Kahan A, Weber S, Amor B, et al. Nifedipine in the treatment of migraine in patients with Raynand's phenomenon. N Engl J Med 1983; 308:1102–1103.

by 58 percent in the flunarizine group. With regard to adverse effects, drowsiness was equally common in both groups, but tachycardia was more common in the nifedipine group.

Nifedipine was compared with propranolol in an open, *parallel* study.[53] The trial involved 40 patients, 20 of whom completed the study. The dose of nifedipine was 20 mg three times per day; the propranolol dose was 40 mg three times per day. The treatment periods were six months in duration. In comparison to the pretrial condition, the frequency of the headaches decreased in the nifedipine group by 25 percent during the first three months of treatment and by 58 percent during the last three months (Figure 5.7). In the propranolol group, the decrease was 62 percent during the first three months of treatment and 64 percent during the last three months. Adverse effects were experienced by *all* patients in the nifedipine group and by 83 percent of the patients in the propranolol group.

Nimodipine

Nimodipine (Nimotop, UK/US) was studied in five double-blind, placebo-controlled trials. The two largest studies are reviewed here; both used the same protocol: They were *parallel* studies with treatment periods of 12 weeks in duration, preceded by a baseline period of four weeks. The dose of the medication was 40 mg three times per day. The first trial involved 192 patients with common migraine or migraine without aura, 161 of whom completed the study.[54] The number of days with migraine decreased by 33 percent from baseline in the nimodipine group and by 35 percent in the placebo group. Adverse effects were equally common in both groups.

The second trial involved 89 patients with classic migraine or migraine with aura, 72 of whom completed the study.[55] The number of days with migraine decreased by 53 percent from baseline in the nimodipine group and by 71 percent in the placebo group. Again, adverse effects were equally common in both groups.

Nimodipine was compared with pizotifen in a double-blind, *crossover* study.[56] The trial involved 43 patients, 36 of whom completed the study. The dose of nimodipine was 40 mg three times per day; the pizotifen dose was 0.5 mg three times per day. The treatment periods were 12 weeks in duration, preceded by a *placebo* baseline period of four weeks. The frequency of the attacks decreased by 52 percent from baseline during treatment with nimodipine and by 29 percent during treatment with pizotifen. The duration of the attacks decreased by 11 and 5 percent from baseline, respectively. Sixty-five percent of the patients experienced an improvement of 50 percent or more in their migraine condition during treatment with nimodipine and 60 percent during treatment with pizotifen. Adverse effects were only experienced during treatment with pizotifen and consisted of weight gain, fatigue, lightheadedness, and nausea.

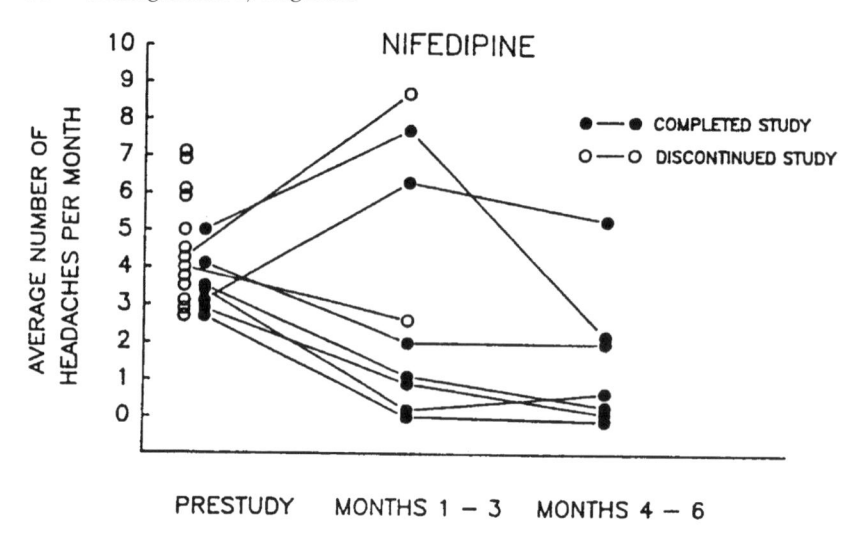

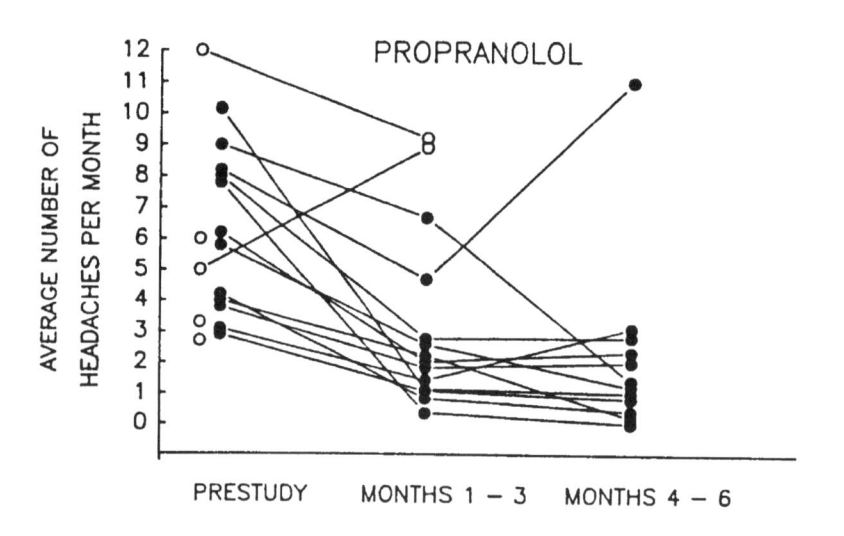

FIGURE 5.7 Effects of nifedipine, 20 mg three times per day, and propranolol, 40 mg three times per day, on the average number of headaches per month. From Albers GW, Simon LT, Hamik A, Peroutka SJ. Nifedipine versus propranolol for the initial prophylaxis of migraine. Headache 1989; 29:214–217 with permission.

Verapamil

Verapamil (Cordilox, UK; Isoptin, US) was studied in two double-blind, placebo-controlled, *crossover* trials. The first trial involved 23 patients, 12 of whom completed the study.[57] The dose of the medication was 80 mg four times per day. The treatment periods were three months in duration. The frequency of the attacks was 43 percent lower during treatment with verapamil than during placebo treatment. No adverse effects occurred during treatment with verapamil except for hypotension in one patient.

The second trial involved 28 patients, 14 of whom completed the study.[58] The dose of the medication was 80 mg three times per day. The treatment periods were eight weeks in duration. The frequency and duration of the headaches were 18 percent lower during treatment with verapamil than during placebo treatment. With regard to adverse effects, 43 percent of the patients experienced constipation during treatment with verapamil.

Miscellaneous Medications

The miscellaneous medications that are effective in the preventive treatment of migraine are clonidine and valproate. Clonidine is an antihypertensive and valproate an antiepileptic medication. A summary of the reported efficacies of clonidine is presented in Table 5.10 and of valproate in Table 5.11.

Clonidine

Clonidine (Catapres, UK/US) was studied in seven double-blind, placebo-controlled, *crossover* trials, the three largest of which are reviewed here. The first trial involved 71 patients, 49 of whom completed the study.[59] The dose of the medication was 0.05 mg two times per day. The treatment periods were eight weeks in duration. The number of attacks was identical during treatment with clonidine and during placebo treatment. The duration of the attacks was 18 percent lower during treatment with clonidine than during placebo treatment. Adverse effects were experienced by 26 percent of the patients during treatment with clonidine and by 12 percent during placebo treatment.

TABLE 5.10
Reported efficacies of clonidine in the preventive treatment of migraine

Dose	Efficacy	Study
0.05 mg/day	25 percent decrease in attack frequency from baseline	Shafar et al., 1972[61]
0.075 mg/day	43 percent decrease in attack frequency from pretrial condition	Kallanranta et al., 1977[60]
0.1 mg/day	5 percent decrease in attack frequency from *placebo* baseline	Louis et al., 1985[63]

TABLE 5.11
Reported efficacies of valproate in the preventive treatment of migraine

Dose	Efficacy	Study
800 mg/day	Attack frequency 43 percent lower than during placebo treatment	Hering & Kuritzky, 1992[64]
1,000–1,500 mg/day	43 percent decrease in the number of migraine days from baseline	Jensen et al., 1994[66]
1,087 mg/day	42 percent decrease in migraine frequency from *placebo* baseline	Mathew et al., 1995[65]

The second trial involved 50 patients, all of whom completed the study.[60] The dose of the medication was 0.025 mg three times per day. The treatment periods were one month in duration. In comparison to the pretrial condition, the frequency of the attacks decreased by 43 percent during treatment with clonidine and by 24 percent during placebo treatment. The duration of the attacks decreased by 44 percent during treatment with clonidine and by 13 percent during placebo treatment. Adverse effects were experienced by 14 percent of the patients during treatment with clonidine and by 14 percent during placebo treatment.

The third trial involved 65 patients, 42 of whom completed the study.[61] The dose of the medication was 0.025 mg two times per day. The treatment periods were 16 weeks in duration, preceded by a baseline period of one month. The frequency of the attacks decreased by 25 percent from baseline during treatment with clonidine and by 17 percent during placebo treatment. Adverse effects were experienced by 40 percent of the patients during treatment with clonidine and by 21 percent during placebo treatment. The most common adverse effects during treatment with clonidine were gastrointestinal upset, dry mouth, and anxiety.

Clonidine was compared with propranolol in a double-blind, *crossover* study.[62] The trial involved 23 patients, 21 of whom completed the study. The dose of clonidine was 0.05 mg two times per day; the propranolol dose was 80 mg two times per day. The treatment periods were 16 weeks in duration of which the first four weeks were excluded from the analysis. The number of days with headache was the same during treatment with clonidine as during treatment with propranolol. In comparison to the pretrial condition, 38 percent of the patients improved more than 50 percent during treatment with clonidine and 62 percent during treatment with propranolol. Adverse effects were experienced by 52 percent of the patients during treatment with clonidine and by 62 percent during treatment with propranolol. The most common adverse effect during treatment with clonidine was fatigue. During treatment with propranolol, the most common adverse effects were lightheadedness, insomnia, and fatigue.

Clonidine was compared with metoprolol in a double-blind, *crossover* study.[63] The trial involved 31 patients, 23 of whom completed the study. The dose of clonidine was 0.05 mg two times per day; the metoprolol dose was 50 mg two times per day. The treatment periods were eight weeks in duration, preceded by a *placebo* baseline period of four weeks. The frequency of the attacks decreased by 5 percent from baseline during treatment with clonidine and by 31 percent during treatment with metoprolol. The number of days with headache decreased by 8 percent from baseline during treatment with clonidine and by 40 percent during treatment with metoprolol. In comparison to baseline, 30 percent of the patients experienced a more than 50 percent reduction in headache days during treatment with clonidine and 37 percent during treatment with metoprolol. Adverse effects were experienced by 41 percent of the patients during treatment with clonidine and by 41 percent during treatment with metoprolol.

Valproate

Valproate (Epilim, UK; Depakote, US) was studied in three double-blind, placebo-controlled trials. The first was a *crossover* trial and involved 32 patients, 29 of whom completed the study.[64] The dose of the medication was 400 mg two times per day. The treatment periods were eight weeks in duration. The frequency of the attacks was 43 percent lower during treatment with valproate than during placebo treatment (Figure 5.8). The intensity of the attacks was 39 percent lower and the duration 38 percent shorter. Adverse effects were experienced by 21 percent of the patients during treatment with valproate and by 7 percent during placebo treatment. The adverse effects experienced during treatment with valproate were indigestion, nausea, and fatigue.

The second was also a *crossover* trial and involved 43 patients, 34 of whom completed the study.[65] The dose of the medication was 1,000 or 1,500 mg per day. The treatment periods were 12 weeks in duration, preceded by a *placebo baseline* period of four weeks. The number of days with migraine decreased by 43 percent from baseline during treatment with valproate and by 0 percent during placebo treatment. Fifty percent of the patients experienced a reduction in migraine days of 50 percent or more during treatment with valproate and 18 percent during placebo treatment. The intensity and duration of the attacks were not affected by the treatments. Adverse effects were experienced by 32 percent of the patients during treatment with valproate and by 16 percent during placebo treatment. The most common adverse effects during treatment with valproate were drowsiness, nausea, lightheadedness, weight gain, and abdominal pain.

The third was a *parallel* trial and involved 117 patients, 105 of whom completed the study.[66] The treatment periods were 12 weeks in duration,

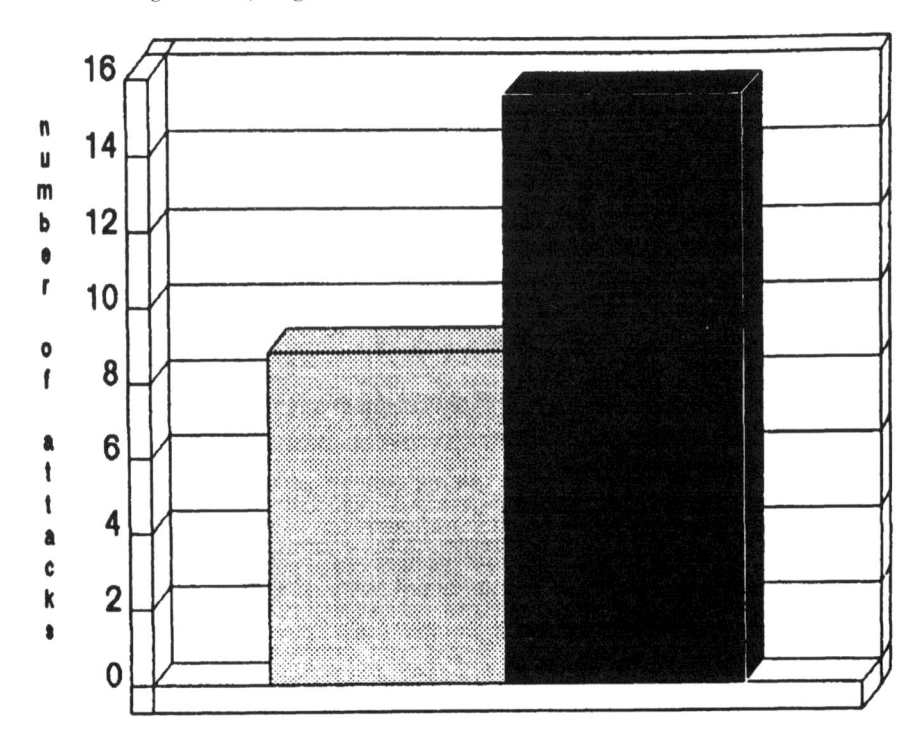

FIGURE 5.8 Number of migraine attacks during eight weeks of treatment with valproate, 400 mg two times per day (gray column), and placebo (black column). From Hering R, Kuritzky A. Sodium valproate in the prophylactic treatment of migraine: A double-blind study versus placebo. Cephalalgia 1992; 12:81–84 with permission.

preceded by a *placebo* baseline period of four weeks. The dose of the medication was adjusted during the first four weeks of treatment to achieve valproate-sodium plasma concentrations of approximately 70 to 120 mg/liter. The mean dose of the medication during the treatment period was 1,087 mg per day; the mean plasma concentration was 66 mg/liter. The frequency of migraine headaches decreased by 42 percent from baseline during treatment with divalproex sodium and by 11 percent during placebo treatment. Of the patients treated with the medication, 48 percent experienced a reduction in frequency of migraine headaches of 50 percent or more from baseline, as compared to 14 percent of those treated with placebo. There were no changes in intensity or duration of the migraine headaches in either treatment group. With regard to adverse effects, nausea was experienced by 46 percent of the patients treated with divalproex sodium and by 14 percent of those treated with placebo. Asthenia was experience by 31 and 8 percent, respectively, and drowsiness by 30 and 5 percent, respectively.

Efficacy

With regard to the efficacy of the preventive antimigraine medications, a summary of rounded estimates is presented in Table 5.12. When compared with placebo, the estimated efficacies are based on an assumed placebo response of 20 percent. The efficacies of the preventive antimigraine medications range from 30 to 70 percent. However, most of the preventive antimigraine medications listed have estimated efficacies that lie between 50 and 60 percent in reducing the frequency of migraine attacks. Exceptions are ergotamine, aspirin, and clonidine, which seem to have much lower efficacies, i.e., around 30 to 40 percent.

The ergot alkaloids and anti-inflammatory medications have a relatively rapid onset of action while at the same time, generally, they are not tolerated well long-term. The ergot alkaloids are not tolerated well long-term because of their vasoconstrictor action, and the anti-inflammatory

TABLE 5.12
Preventive antimigraine medications with rounded estimates of their efficacy*

Medication	Efficacy
Ergot alkaloids	
Ergotamine (0.6 mg two times per day)	35 percent
Methysergide (6 mg per day)	55 percent
Serotonin antagonists	
Pizotifen (1.5 to 3 mg per day)	50 percent
Beta-receptor blockers	
Atenolol (100 mg per day)	50 percent
Metoprolol (100 to 200 mg per day)	50 percent
Nadolol (80 to 240 mg per day)	70 percent
Propranolol (80 to 160 mg per day)	55 percent
Timolol (10 mg two times per day)	50 percent
Tricyclic antidepressants	
Amitriptyline (10 to 150 mg per day)	60 percent
Anti-inflammatory medications	
Aspirin (1,000 to 1,500 mg per day)	40 percent
Naproxen sodium (275 to 550 mg two times per day)	60 percent
Calcium-entry blockers	
Flunarizine (10 mg once daily)	50 percent
Nifedipine (20 to 60 mg per day)	60 percent
Nimodipine (40 mg three times per day)	50 percent
Verapamil (80 mg three to four times per day)	50 percent
Miscellaneous medications	
Clonidine (0.05 to 0.1 mg per day)	30 percent
Valproate (800 to 1,500 mg per day)	55 percent

*Medications included only when at least two studies are available.

medications are similarly limited because of their gastrotoxic effect. Therefore, they are best used for short-term migraine prevention (i.e., when migraine attacks occur at predictable times) such as during menstruation, on weekends, during stressful periods, etc. An additional problem with the long-term use of methysergide is the occurrence of such fibrotic conditions as retroperitoneal fibrosis (*vide infra*).

The medications in the remaining five groups generally are tolerated well long-term, although they certainly have their adverse effects. The adverse effects should always be weighed against the beneficial effects of the medications, which generally do not exceed 60 percent in reducing the frequency, intensity, and duration of the attacks. With the exception of nifedipine, the calcium-entry blockers and clonidine generally are tolerated best with least adverse effects. Nifedipine is a relatively potent vasodilator and, consequently, often causes headache, hypotension, and tachycardia. The other calcium-entry blockers are tolerated relatively well. Flunarizine can cause drowsiness, weight gain, and occasionally depression, and verapamil can cause constipation. Clonidine sometimes causes gastrointestinal upset or a dry mouth. The beta-receptor blockers, in particular propranolol, often cause more adverse effects. Propranolol is notorious for causing lethargy, fatigue, depression, insomnia, and impotence. The other beta-blockers generally are tolerated better but still frequently cause fatigue, though to a lesser extent. The serotonin antagonists and amitriptyline often cause drowsiness, dry mouth, constipation, and increased appetite, which can lead to considerable weight gain. Valproate can upset the stomach to cause indigestion and nausea.

Short-Term Prevention

As previously mentioned, the ergot alkaloids and anti-inflammatory analgesics are best used for short-term prevention as they have a relatively rapid onset of action. They also generally are not well tolerated when used for a prolonged period of time.

Short-term prevention has to be initiated at least one or two days before the expected migraine attack. Bellergal-S can be used in a dose of one tablet once or twice daily. When used once daily, the medication is best given at bedtime. With the use of an additional tablet in the morning, drowsiness can occur. Dry mouth and constipation rarely occur as adverse effects of Bellergal.

Dihydroergotamine can be used in a dose of 5 mg once or twice daily. The medication can cause nausea, especially during the first days of treatment. The dose of methysergide ranges from 1 mg four times per day or 2 mg two times per day to 2 mg four times per day. The medication has to be given in two to four divided doses because of its short plasma half-life. It often causes stomach upset with indigestion or nausea, but these adverse effects can be mitigated by taking the medication with meals and at bedtime with food. With intermittent use of the methysergide for short-term prevention, potential fibrotic adverse effects are not a concern. These adverse effects are relevant with prolonged use of the medication for long-term migraine prevention (*vide infra*).

Long-Term Prevention

For the long-term preventive treatment of migraine, the beta-receptor blockers generally are reasonably effective and well tolerated. Propranolol most commonly is used, although it probably has most adverse effects. It is a good medication for patients who are in good physical and mental condition. It can be given once daily when the long-acting preparation is used, but otherwise has to be given in two divided doses. Propranolol can be initiated in a dose of 80 mg per day, which if necessary can be increased with increments of 40 mg. The medication is usually effective in doses between 80 and 160 mg per day. However, if necessary the dose can be further increased until the pulse rate is between 50 and 60 beats per minute. Common adverse effects of propranolol are lethargy, fatigue, depression, insomnia, and impotence. The other beta-blockers generally are tolerated better, although they often still cause fatigue.

Atenolol, metoprolol, and nadolol can be given once daily, whereas timolol has to be given in two divided doses. Atenolol can be initiated in a dose of 50 mg per day, which if necessary can be increased with increments of 50 mg. The medication is usually effective in doses between 50 and 100 mg per day. Metoprolol can be initiated in a dose of 100 mg per day, which if necessary can be increased with increments of 50 mg. The medication is usually effective in doses between 100 and 200 mg per day. Nadolol can be initiated in a dose of 40 mg per day, which if necessary can be increased with increments of 40 mg. The medication is usually effective in doses between 80 and 160 mg per day. Timolol can be initiated in a dose of 20 mg per day, which if necessary can be increased with increments of 10 mg. The medication is usually effective in doses between 20 and 40 mg per day.

Atenolol and metoprolol are $beta_1$-selective or cardioselective but should still be used with great care in patients with obstructive pulmonary disease, including asthma. The beta-blockers also should be used with great care in patients with diabetes mellitus (as they can mask the symptoms of hypoglycemia) and in patients with depression, which can be aggravated by the medications. Furthermore, they should never be stopped abruptly but be tapered gradually. Finally, if a patient does not tolerate a particular beta-blocker, others certainly can be tried. The beta-blockers are contraindicated in patients with sinus bradycardia, obstructive pulmonary disease, atrioventricular block, or congestive heart failure.

In patients who do not sleep well at night and often feel tired as a result, amitriptyline, pizotifen, or cyproheptadine are the first choice. These medications are long-acting and, therefore, can be given once daily. They should be taken at bedtime as they cause drowsiness, which generally assists in inducing sleep in patients who do not sleep well at night. Patients who do sleep well at night often experience day-time drowsiness from the medications, even if they are taken at bedtime. In these patients, the medications generally are tolerated better when they are taken one or two hours *before* bedtime.

Amitriptyline can be initiated in a dose of 25 mg per day, which if necessary can be increased with increments of 25 mg. The medication is usually effective in doses between 25 and 75 mg per day. However, if necessary the dose can be further increased until some dryness of the mouth occurs. Another common adverse effect of amitriptyline is constipation. Pizotifen can be initiated in a dose of 1.5 mg per day, which if necessary can be increased with increments of 0.5 mg. The medication is usually effective in doses between 1.5 and 3 mg per day. Cyproheptadine can be initiated in a dose of 12 mg per day, which if necessary can be increased with increments of 4 mg. The medication is usually effective in doses between 12 and 20 mg per day. Pizotifen and cyproheptadine also cause dry mouth and constipation as adverse effects but to a lesser extent than amitriptyline. However, all three medications stimulate appetite and can cause weight gain. Patients should be warned about this adverse effect, as weight gain is more easily prevented than reversed. The medications are contraindicated in patients with glaucoma, prostate hypertrophy, epilepsy, or cardiac arrhythmias.

As it is an antidepressant, amitriptyline is a good medication for patients who also suffer from depression. However, in these patients the medication should be used in higher doses to obtain the antidepressant effect. The beta-blockers, as well as flunarizine and clonidine, should be used with great care in patients with depression, as they can aggravate the condition. Flunarizine and clonidine do not have other contraindications and generally are tolerated well. Flunarizine causes mild drowsiness and sometimes weight gain. It can be given once daily, as it is a long-acting medication. The dose is 10 mg, preferably taken at bedtime. Clonidine sometimes causes mild drowsiness or a dry mouth. It has to be given in two divided doses per day. The dose for the preventive treatment of migraine is 0.1 or 0.2 mg per day.

Of the remaining calcium-entry blockers, nimodipine and verapamil also generally are tolerated well. The most common adverse effect of verapamil is constipation, and sometimes impotence or male infertility. The medications are contraindicated in patients with sick sinus syndrome or atrioventricular block. The dose of nimodipine is 30 mg four times per day, and that of verapamil is 80 mg four times per day. If necessary, the dose of verapamil can be increased further to 120 mg four times per day. The medication can be given two times per day when the sustained-release preparation is used.

Valproate is not tolerated very well and often causes stomach upset with indigestion or nausea. These adverse effects can be decreased by taking the medication with meals, either two or three times per day. Valproate can be initiated in a dose of 250 mg per day, which if necessary can be increased with increments of 250 mg. The medication is usually effective in doses between 500 and 1,000 mg per day. The serum level can be determined and preferably should be maintained between 50 and 100 ml. The liver function also should be determined regularly because of hepatotoxicity. The medication is contraindicated in patients with abnormal liver function or liver disease.

Methysergide also generally is not tolerated well and often causes stomach upset in addition to indigestion or nausea. Therefore, preferably it also should be taken with meals and at bedtime with food. It has to be given in two or four divided doses because of its short, plasma half-life. Methysergide can be initiated in a dose of 4 mg per day, which if necessary can be increased with increments of 2 mg. The medication is usually effective in doses between 4 and 8 mg per day.

When used long-term, methysergide can cause fibrotic conditions.[67] Most common is retroperitoneal fibrosis with the formation of fibrotic tissue in the retroperitoneal space. Less common are pleuropulmonary and endocardial fibrosis. Retroperitoneal fibrosis manifests itself through pain in the abdomen or back and swelling of the leg(s). The pain in the abdomen and back are caused by hydronephrosis due to obstruction of the ureter(s). The swelling of the leg(s) is caused by obstruction of the inferior vena cava. Pleuropulmonary fibrosis manifests itself through chest pain and shortness of breath. Endocardial fibrosis generally remains asymptomatic but is characterized by the development of heart murmurs. The fibrotic conditions can be prevented by interrupting the treatment with methysergide for one month every four to six months. The medication is contraindicated in patients with hypertension, coronary artery disease, peripheral vascular disease, valvular heart disease, pulmonary disease, collagen vascular disease, or fibrotic conditions.

The suggested sequence of use of the preventive antimigraine medications for short- and long-term migraine prevention is summarized in Table 5.13. The medications can be used individually but also can be combined. However, an attempt should always be made first to obtain satisfactory prevention with a single medication. When a medication is insufficiently effective or its dose cannot be further increased because of adverse effects, the addition of a second medication may be considered.

Medications that work well in combination are the beta-blockers and amitriptyline or pizotifen. Amitriptyline and pizotifen also can be combined with flunarizine or clonidine. The beta-blockers should be used with great care in combination with flunarizine because of possible depression as an adverse effect. The beta-blockers should *not* be combined with clonidine because of the risk of causing hypotension and depression. They should also not be combined with the other calcium-entry blockers because of the risk of causing hypotension and bradycardia.

TABLE 5.13
Summary of preventive migraine treatment

Short-term prevention
   Dihydroergotamine, ergotamine (Bellergal), or methysergide
   Naproxen sodium
Long-term prevention
   First choice: propranolol, atenolol, metoprolol, nadolol, or timolol
   Second choice: amitriptyline, pizotifen, or flunarizine
   Third choice: verapamil or nimodipine
   Forth choice: valproate or methysergide
   Fifth choice: aspirin, clonidine, cyproheptadine, or nifedipine

Amitriptyline, pizotifen, and flunarizine should not be used in combination because they can cause weight gain. However, amitriptyline and pizotifen can be combined with the other calcium-entry blockers. Finally, methysergide should not be combined with the beta-blockers because of the potential for peripheral vasoconstriction.

Mode of Action

The ergot alkaloids directly address two important aspects of the pathogenesis of the migraine headache: arterial vasodilation and neurogenic inflammation. The mechanism of neurogenic inflammation also is addressed by the anti-inflammatory medications. The beta-blockers that are effective in the preventive treatment of migraine share a lack of partial agonist or intrinsic sympathomimetic activity (Table 5.14). This means that they increase peripheral vascular resistance by increasing blood vessel tone. The increased blood vessel tone hampers the dilation of the extracranial arteries, thereby

TABLE 5.14
Pharmacological features of the beta-receptor blockers effective in the preventive treatment of migraine

	Cardio-selective	Partial agonist	Membrane stabilizing	Lipid soluble
Atenolol	Yes	No	No	No
Metoprolol	Yes	No	No	No
Nadolol	No	No	No	No
Propranolol	No	No	Yes	Yes
Timolol	No	No	No	Yes

preventing migraine attacks. Amitriptyline potentiates the effects of serotonin in the central nervous system by blocking its re-uptake. Serotonin inhibits the transmission of pain signals in the central nervous system, thereby increasing the pain threshold.

Pizotifen and cyproheptadine may prevent migraine attacks through a mechanism similar to that of amitriptyline. Though they are traditionally known as serotonin antagonists, they potentiate the effects of serotonin in low concentrations. This may be relevant to their effects in the central nervous system which is, to a great extent, protected from the penetration of medications by the blood-brain barrier. The calcium-entry blockers also have been shown recently to increase the pain threshold.[68] This was more pronounced for nimodipine than for verapamil, an effect that was related to the higher lipid solubility of the former. The effect of the calcium-entry blockers on the pain threshold is attributed to an impairment of synaptic transmission at the level of the spinal cord.

Clonidine reduces vascular reactivity, the mechanism implicated in migraine prevention. The mechanism of action of valproate in the preventive treatment of migraine is not known.

References

1. Stieg RL. Double-blind study of belladonna-ergotamine-phenobarbital for the interval treatment of recurrent throbbing headache. Headache 1977; 17:120–124.
2. Curran DA, Lance JW. Clinical trial of methysergide and other preparations in the management of migraine. J Neurol Neurosurg Psychiatry 1964; 27:463–469.
3. Neuman M, Demarez JP, Harmey JL, et al. Prevention of migraine attacks through the use of dihydroergotamine. Int J Clin Pharmacol Res 1986; 6:11–13.
4. Shekelle RB, Ostfeld AM. Methysergide in the migraine syndrome. Clin Pharmacol Ther 1964; 5:201–204.
5. Southwell N, Williams JD, MacKenzie I. Methysergide in the prophylaxis of migraine. Lancet 1964; 1:523–524.
6. Pedersen E, Moller CE. Methysergide in migraine prophylaxis. Clin Pharmacol Ther 1966; 4:520–526.
7. Arthur GP, Hornabrook RW. The treatment of migraine with BC 105 (pizotifen): A double-blind trial. N Z Med J 1971; 73:5–9.
8. Andersson PG. BC-105 and Deseril in migraine prophylaxis (a double-blind study). Headache 1973; 13:68–73.
9. Diamond S, Medina J. Double-blind study of propranolol for migraine prophylaxis. Headache 1976; 16:24–27.
10. Nadelmann JW, Stevens J, Saper JR. Propranolol in the prophylaxis of migraine. Headache 1986; 26:175–182.
11. Havanka-Kanniainen H, Hokkanen E, Myllyla VV. Long-acting propranolol in the prophylaxis of migraine. Comparison of the daily doses of 80 mg and 160 mg. Headache 1988; 28:607–611.

12. Carroll JD, Reidy M, Savundra P, et al. Long-acting propranolol in the prophylaxis of migraine: A comparative study of two doses. Cephalalgia 1990; 10:101–105.
13. Behan PO, Reid M. Propranolol in the treatment of migraine. Practitioner 1980; 224:201–204.
14. Johannsson V, Nilsson LR, Widelius T, et al. Atenolol in migraine prophylaxis. A double-blind cross-over multicentre study. Headache 1987; 27:372–374.
15. Forssman B, Lindblad CJ, Zbornikova V. Atenolol for migraine prophylaxis. Headache 1983; 23:188–190.
16. Stensrud P, Sjaastad O. Comparative trial of Tenormin (atenolol) and Inderal (propranolol) in migraine. Headache 1980; 20:204–207.
17. Andersson PG, Dahl S, Hansen JH, et al. Prophylactic treatment of classical and non-classical migraine with metoprolol—A comparison with placebo. Cephalalgia 1983; 3:207–212.
18. Olsson JE, Behring HC, Forssman B, et al. Metoprolol and propranolol in migraine prophylaxis: A double-blind multicentre study. Acta Neurol Scand 1984; 70:160–168.
19. Kangasniemi P, Hedman C. Metoprolol and propranolol in the prophylactic treatment of classical and common migraine. A double-blind study. Cephalalgia 1984; 4:91–96.
20. Vilming S, Standnes B, Hedman C. Metoprolol and pizotifen in the prophylactic treatment of classical and common migraine. A double-blind investigation. Cephalalgia 1985; 5:17–23.
21. Ryan RE, Ryan RE, Sudilovsky A. Nadolol: Its use in the prophylactic treatment of migraine. Headache 1983; 23:26–31.
22. Sudilovsky A, Elkind A, Ryan RE, et al. Comparative efficacy of nadolol and propranolol in the management of migraine. Headache 1987; 27:421–426.
23. Ryan RE. Comparative study of nadolol and propranolol in prophylactic treatment of migraine. Am Heart J 1984; 108:1156–1159.
24. Stellar S, Ahrens SP, Meibohm AR, Reines SA. Migraine prevention with timolol. A double-blind crossover study. JAMA 1984; 252:2576–2580.
25. Tfelt-Hansen P, Standnes B, Kangasniemi P, et al. Timolol vs propranolol vs placebo in common migraine prophylaxis: A double-blind multicenter trial. Acta Neurol Scand 1984; 69:18.
26. Gomersall JD, Stuart A. Amitriptyline in migraine prophylaxis. Changes in pattern of attacks during a controlled clinical trial. J Neurol Neurosurg Psychiatry 1973; 36:684–690.
27. Couch JR, Hassanein RS. Amitriptyline in migraine prophylaxis. Arch Neurol 1979; 36:695–699.
28. Ziegler DK, Hurwitz A, Hassanein RS, et al. Migraine prophylaxis. A comparison of propranolol and amitriptyline. Arch Neurol 1987; 44:486–489.
29. Ziegler DK, Hurwitz A, Preskorn S, et al. Propranolol and amitriptyline in prophylaxis of migraine. Pharmacokinetic and therapeutic effects. Arch Neurol 1993; 50:825–830.
30. Bank J. A comparative study of amitriptyline and fluvoxamine in migraine prophylaxis. Headache 1994; 34:476–478.
31. Saper JR, Silberstein SD, Lake AE, et al. Double-blind trial of fluoxetine: Chronic daily headache and migraine. Headache 1994; 34:497–502.

32. Noone JF. Clomipramine in the prevention of migraine. J Intern Med Res 1980; 8 (suppl 3):49–52.
33. Langohr HD, Gerber WD, Koletzki E, et al. Clomipramine and metoprolol in migraine prophylaxis—A double-blind crossover study. Headache 1985; 25:107–113.
34. O'Neill BP, Mann JD. Aspirin prophylaxis in migraine. Lancet 1978; 2:1179–1181.
35. Buring JE, Peto R, Hennekens CH. Low-dose aspirin for migraine prophylaxis. JAMA 1990; 264:1711–1713.
36. Baldrati A, Cortelli P, Procaccianti G, et al. Propranolol and acetylsalicylic acid in migraine prophylaxis. Double-blind crossover study. Acta Neurol Scand 1983; 67:181–186.
37. Grotemeyer KH, Scharafinsky HW, Schlake HP, Husstedt IW. Acetylsalicylic acid versus metoprolol in migraine prophylaxis—A double-blind cross-over study. Headache 1990; 30:639–641.
38. Welch KMA, Ellis DJ, Keenan PA. Successful migraine prophylaxis with naproxen sodium. Neurology 1985; 35:1304–1310.
39. Ziegler DK, Ellis DJ. Naproxen in prophylaxis of migraine. Arch Neurol 1985; 42:582–584.
40. Sargent J, Solbach P, Damasio H, et al. A comparison of naproxen sodium to propranolol hydrochloride and a placebo control for the prophylaxis of migraine headache. Headache 1985; 25:320–324.
41. Bellavance AJ, Meloche JP. A comparative study of naproxen sodium, pizotyline and placebo in migraine prophylaxis. Headache 1990; 30:710–715.
42. Mikkelsen BM, Falk JV. Prophylactic treatment of migraine with tolfenamic acid. Acta Neurol Scand 1982; 66:105–111.
43. Diamond S, Solomon GD, Freitag FG, Mehta ND. Fenoprofen in the prophylaxis of migraine: A double-blind, placebo controlled study. Headache 1987; 27:246–249.
44. Anthony M, Lance JW. Indomethacin in migraine. Med J Aust 1968; 1:56–57.
45. Louis P. A double-blind placebo-controlled prophylactic study of flunarizine (Sibelium) in migraine. Headache 1981; 21:235–239.
46. Soelberg Sorensen P, Hansen K, Olesen J. A placebo-controlled, double-blind, cross-over trial of flunarizine in common migraine. Cephalalgia 1986; 6:7–14.
47. Spierings ELH, Messinger HB. Flunarizine vs. pizotifen in migraine prophylaxis: A review of comparative studies. Cephalalgia 1988; 8 (suppl 8):27–30.
48. Ludin HP. Flunarizine and propranolol in the treatment of migraine. Headache 1989; 29:218–223.
49. Soelberg Sorensen P, Larsen BH, Rasmussen MJK, et al. Flunarizine versus metoprolol in migraine prophylaxis: A double-blind, randomized parallel group study of efficacy and tolerability. Headache 1991; 31:650–657.
50. Leandri M, Rigardo S, Schizzi R, Parodi CI. Migraine treatment with nicardipine. Cephalalgia 1990; 10:111–116.
51. Kahan A, Weber S, Amor B, et al. Nifedipine in the treatment of migraine in patients with Raynaud's phenomenon. N Engl J Med 1983; 308:1102–1103.
52. Lamsudin R, Sadjimin T. Comparison of the efficacy between flunarizine and nifedipine in the prophylaxis of migraine. Headache 1993; 33:335–338.
53. Albers GW, Simon LT, Hamik A, Peroutka SJ. Nifedipine versus propranolol for the initial prophylaxis of migraine. Headache 1989; 29:214–217.

54. Migraine-Nimodipine European Study Group. European multicenter trial of nimodipine in the prophylaxis of common migraine (migraine without aura). Headache 1989; 29:633–638.
55. Migraine-Nimodipine European Study Group. European multicenter trial of nimodipine in the prophylaxis of classic migraine (migraine with aura). Headache 1989; 29:639–642.
56. Havanka-Kanniainen H, Hokkanen E, Myllyla VV. Efficacy of nimodipine in comparison with pizotifen in the prophylaxis of migraine. Cephalalgia 1987; 7:7–13.
57. Solomon GD, Steel JG, Spaccavento LJ. Verapamil prophylaxis of migraine. A double-blind, placebo-controlled study. JAMA 1983; 250:2500–2502.
58. Markley HG, Cheronis JCD, Piepho RW. Verapamil in the prophylactic therapy of migraine. Neurology 1984; 34:973–976.
59. Boisen E, Deth S, Hubbe P, et al. Clonidine in the prophylaxis of migraine. Acta Neurol Scand 1978; 58:288–295.
60. Kallanranta T, Hakkarainen H, Hokkanen E, Tuovinen T. Clonidine in migraine prophylaxis. Headache 1977; 17:169–172.
61. Shafar J, Tallett ER, Knowlson PA. Evaluation of clonidine in prophylaxis of migraine. Double-blind trial and follow-up. Lancet 1972; 1:403–407.
62. Kass B, Nestvold K. Propranolol (Inderal) and clonidine (Catapressan) in the prophylactic treatment of migraine. A comparative trial. Acta Neurol Scand 1980; 61:351–356.
63. Louis P, Schoenen J, Hedman C. Metoprolol versus clonidine in the prophylactic treatment of migraine. Cephalalgia 1985; 5:159–165.
64. Hering R, Kuritzky A. Sodium valproate in the prophylactic treatment of migraine: A double-blind study versus placebo. Cephalalgia 1992; 12:81–84.
65. Jensen R, Brinck T, Olesen J. Sodium valproate has a prophylactic effect in migraine without aura: A triple-blind, placebo controlled cross-over study. Neurology 1994; 44:647–651.
66. Mathew NT, Saper JR, Silberstein SD, et al. Migraine prophylaxis with divalproex. Arch Neurol 1995; 52:281–286.
67. Graham JR, Suby HI, LeCompte PM, Sadowsky NL. Inflammatory fibrosis associated with methysergide therapy. Res Clin Stud Headache 1967; 1:123–164.
68. Miranda HF, Bustamante D, Kramer V, et al. Antinociceptive effects of Ca^{2+} channel blockers. Eur J Pharmacol 1992; 217:137–141.

CHAPTER 6

Endogenous and Exogenous Trigger Factors

Trigger factors are events that bring on a migraine attack and are endogenous or exogenous in nature. Probably the most potent endogenous trigger factor is the estrogen cycle in women, which largely accounts for the two or three times higher prevalence of migraine in women than in men. An important exogenous trigger factor of migraine is stress; very typically, the attack triggered by stress comes after the stressful event rather than during it. Other exogenous trigger factors of migraine are weather changes, alcoholic beverages, and dietary products. Endogenous trigger factors other than the menstrual cycle in women are fatigue, lack of sleep, oversleeping, and lack of food. The trigger factors often need each other to bring on a migraine attack; therefore, one strategy in reducing the frequency of the attacks is to prevent factors from compounding.

Estrogen Cycle

In women, migraine attacks are particularly likely to occur during *menstruation* and tend to be more severe and long-lasting during this time of the menstrual cycle. In a *diary* study, 74 women who were between 22 and 29 yeas old and 30 percent of whom used oral contraceptives recorded a total of 241 menstrual periods.[1] The risk of migraine without aura, but not that of migraine with aura, was increased by two-thirds during the first three days of menstruation. The risk was not increased during the two days before menstruation (i.e., the premenstrual days) or on the estimated day of ovulation.

In an analysis of 142 migraine-afflicted women attending a migraine clinic, 24 percent experienced the onset of migraine in the same year or the year after menarche (Figure 6.1).[2] Of the 92 women who were still menstruating, 14 percent experienced attacks *only* with menstruation, 12 percent regularly with menstruation but also at other times, 13 percent with some menstrual periods only, and 45 percent sometimes with menstruation but

106 *Management of Migraine*

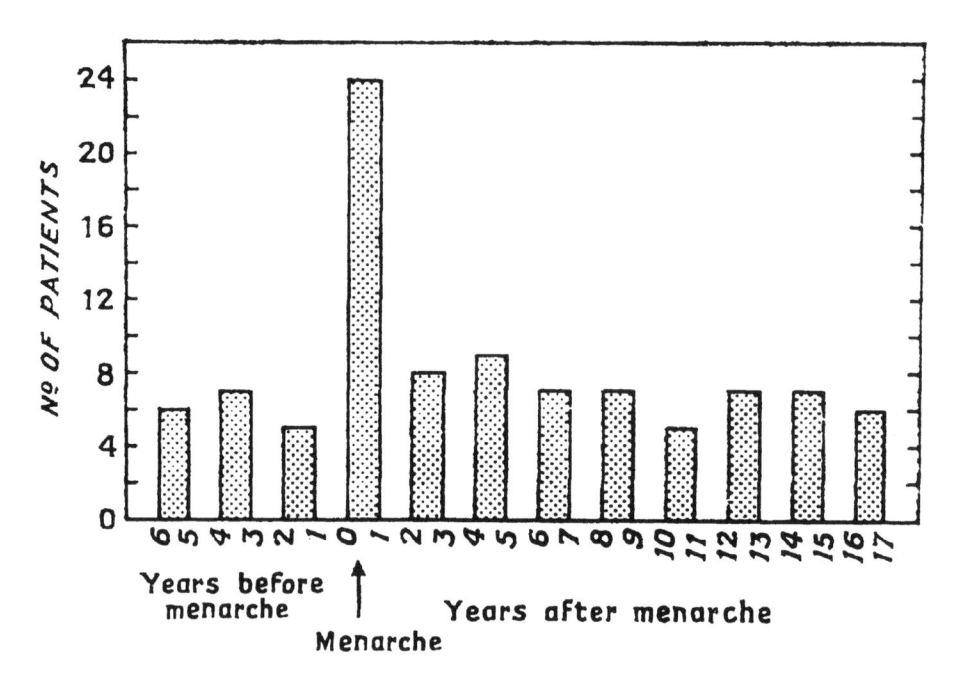

FIGURE 6.1 Age of onset of migraine in relation to menarche, showing the intervals in years between the first attack and the onset of menstruation. From Epstein MT, Hockaday JM, Hockaday TDR. Migraine and reproductive hormones throughout the menstrual cycle. Lancet 1975; 1:543–548 with permission.

also at other times. In the 120 women who experienced migraine attacks while still menstruating, there was an association between the occurrence of attacks during menstruation and menstrual symptoms. The menstrual symptoms considered were weight gain as a symptom of fluid retention and breast discomfort as a symptom of direct hormonal tissue effect. It was found that when both symptoms occur with menstruation, the likelihood of migraine occurring during menstruation is 62 percent, as opposed to 33 percent when both symptoms are absent.

With regard to the effect of *pregnancy*, of the 83 patients who experienced migraine before they ever got pregnant, 66 percent noted improvement, 22 percent noted no change, and 12 percent reported worsening during at least one pregnancy. Of the patients whose migraine had occurred regularly and *only* in relation to menstruation, 90 percent noted an improvement with pregnancy, as opposed to 38 percent of the patients who denied any relationship. With regard to the effect of *menopause* in the women who had ceased menstruating, the likelihood of improvement or worsening of migraine was random either at, or after, menopause.

In a *prospective* study of 484 women with migraine, 17 percent became headache-free during pregnancy, 27 percent improved definitely, 35 percent improved probably, and 21 percent did not improve.[3] The women in the unimproved group were more likely than the others to have had at least four pregnancies and to have had hypertension or so-called pre-eclampsia.

Hormonal studies in women with migraine revealed similar mean plasma levels of luteinizing hormone (LH) and follicle stimulating hormone (FSH) as compared to controls (Figure 6.2).[2] However, the mean plasma levels of the ovarian hormones estrogen and progesterone were significantly higher than in controls (Figure 6.2). With regard to the ovarian hormones, no differences were observed between the women with migraine predominantly before or during menstruation and those with attacks randomly throughout the menstrual cycle.

In relation to the changes in plasma estrogen and progesterone levels, the attacks in women with menstrual migraine occur during the terminal phase of the estrogen and progesterone withdrawal, as is illustrated in Figure 6.3.[4] Treatment with estradiol (thereby artificially maintaining the plasma estrogen level) delayed the migraine attack, though the progesterone withdrawal and menstruation still occurred. Treatment with progesterone had the opposite effect (i.e., it delayed menstruation while the migraine attack nevertheless occurred).[5] Attempts have been made, therefore, to prevent the occurrence of migraine attacks during menstruation by treatment with estradiol.

Estradiol

Estradiol is available as an oral tablet (Progynova, UK; Estrace, US), vaginal cream (Estrace, US), subcutaneous implant (UK), and transdermal patch (Estraderm, UK/US). It is absorbed well but has an extensive presystemic metabolism and a short plasma half-life. It was studied in the preventive treatment of menstrual migraine by subcutaneous implant, percutaneous gel, and transdermal patch.

The implant was studied in an *open* trial of 24 patients with menstrual migraine.[6] The patients experienced attacks regularly, either immediately before or during menstruation. Treatment was initiated with the 100 mg implant, which was subsequently generally decreased to 50 mg. A new implant was inserted, on the average, once every half year. The patients were given cyclical progestogen (i.e., norethisterone 5 mg per day for seven days once per month, to induce regular endometrial shedding). All but one patient experienced improvement of the menstrual migraine. The improvement was complete in 46 percent of the patients and almost complete in 38 percent. The monthly bleedings were usually lighter and less painful than before treatment, although four patients complained of heavier blood loss. No other adverse effects were caused by the treatment.

The percutaneous estradiol gel was studied in a double-blind, placebo-controlled, *crossover* trial.[7] The trial involved 20 patients, 18 of whom completed the study. The patients suffered from menstrual migraine and had regular menstrual cycles. Menstrual migraine was defined as common mi-

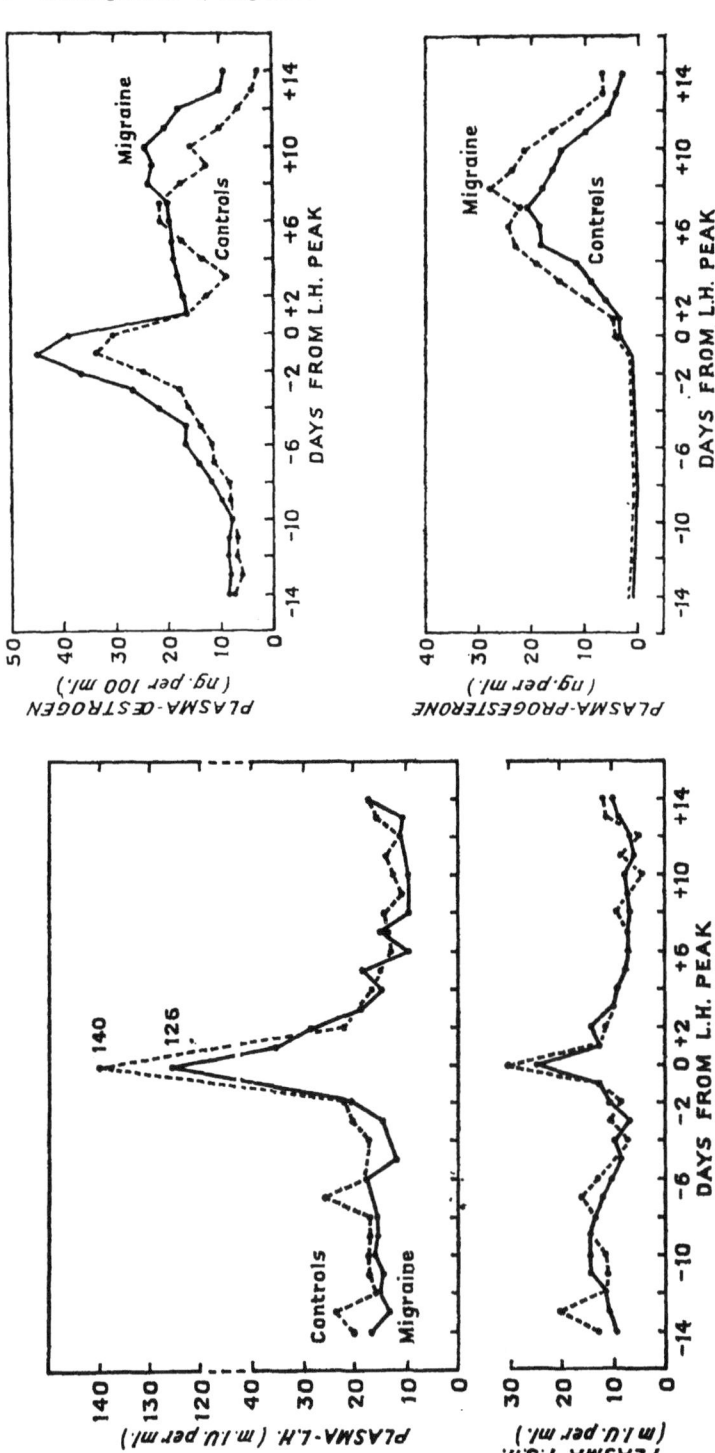

FIGURE 6.2 Means of daily plasma levels of luteinizing hormone (LH), follicle stimulating hormone (FSH; left), estrogen, and progesterone (right) during the menstrual cycle in 14 patients with migraine and 8 controls. From Epstein MT, Hockaday JM, Hockaday TDR. Migraine and reproductive hormones throughout the menstrual cycle. Lancet 1975; 1:543–548 with permission.

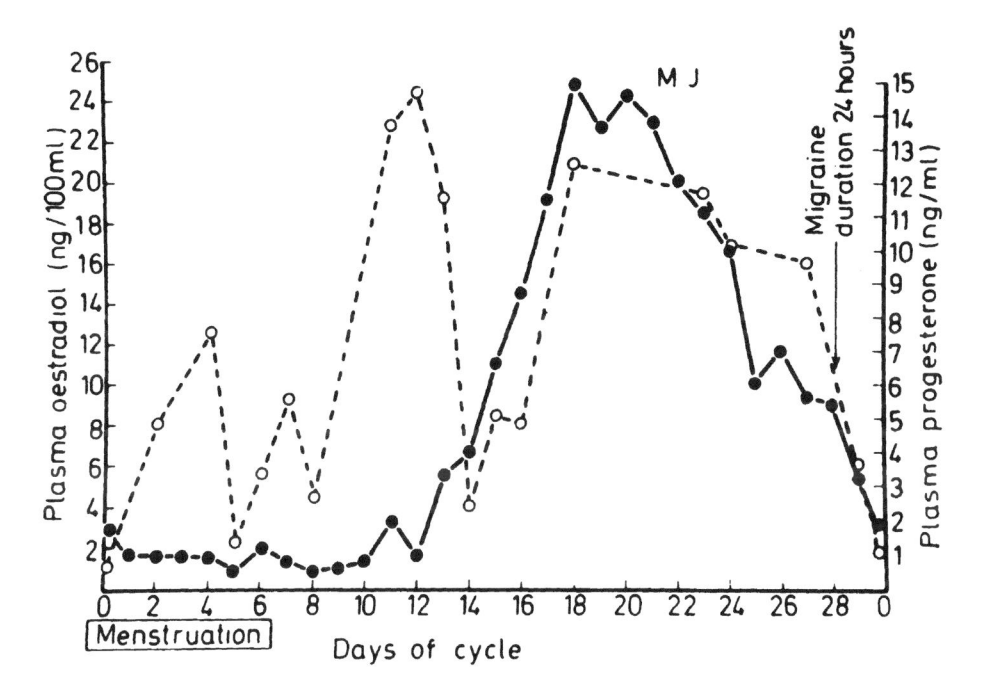

FIGURE 6.3 Daily plasma estradiol and progesterone levels during the menstrual cycle in a woman with menstrual migraine. The arrow indicates the time of onset of the migraine attack. From Somerville BW. The role of estradiol withdrawal in the etiology of menstrual migraine. Neurology 1972; 22:355–365 with permission.

graine or migraine without aura, with the attacks occurring exclusively between two days before and the last day of menstruation. The estradiol preparation contained 1.5 mg estradiol in 2.5 mg gel. The patients applied the gel to the skin daily for seven days each month, starting 48 hours before the earliest expected attack. Menstrual attacks occurred in 31 percent of the cycles treated with estradiol and in 96 percent of those treated with placebo. The attacks that occurred during treatment with estradiol were also considerably less intense and shorter in duration. Changes in the menstrual cycle were observed in 7 percent of the cycles treated with placebo and in 15 percent of those treated with estradiol. Mood changes or breast discomfort did not occur.

The transdermal patch was studied in a placebo-controlled, *crossover* trial.[8] The trial involved 20 patients, all of whom completed the study. The patients suffered from menstrual migraine and had regular menstrual cycles. Menstrual migraine was defined as in the percutaneous gel study described above. The patch delivered 0.05 mg estradiol per day. It was applied 48 hours before the expected onset of menstruation and again four days later. Menstrual attacks occurred in 59 percent of the cycles treated with estradiol and in 69 percent of those treated with placebo. The intensity and duration of the attacks were also not different between the two treatments.

Oral Contraceptives

Oral contraceptives generally contain an estrogen and a progestogen. The estrogens used in the oral contraceptives are ethinyl estradiol or its methyl ether, mestranol. Currently, the oral contraceptives most frequently used contain ethinyl estradiol in a dose of less than 0.05 mg. Ethinyl estradiol is about two hundred times more potent than the above-mentioned estradiol. Oral contraceptives suppress ovulation but do *not* eliminate or alleviate the estrogen cycle. Actually, they cause a more pronounced estrogen withdrawal before the monthly bleeding occurs. Therefore, it is not surprising that oral contraceptives often make migraine (especially menstrual migraine) worse.

Ovral, an oral contraceptive containing 0.05 mg ethinyl estradiol, was studied in an *open, crossover* trial.[9] The trial involved 40 patients, all of whom completed the study. The treatment periods were two months in duration. The number of headaches was 45 percent higher during treatment with the oral contraceptive. The number of mild headaches was 31 percent higher, that of moderate headaches 44 percent, and of severe headaches 60 percent. With regard to the overall migraine condition, 70 percent of the patients were worse on the oral contraceptive, and 30 percent were better.

In a *retrospective* study of 122 female migraine patients who had taken an oral contraceptive, 66 percent were worse on the oral contraceptive, and 34 percent were better.[10] Of the 47 patients with predominantly menstrual attacks, 81 percent were worse as opposed to 57 percent of the 75 patients with random attacks. In a group of 56 patients who used oral contraceptives, 70 percent improved after the oral contraceptives were discontinued.[11] Of the patients who experienced more than four attacks per month, 87 percent improved, and of those who experienced less than one attack per month, 33 percent improved. Improvement was defined as a decrease in frequency of the attacks by at least 60 percent.

An oral contraceptive containing progestogen only was studied in an *open* trial.[12] The trial involved 24 patients, 22 of whom completed the study. The patients took the medication daily without interruptions. The duration of the treatment period ranged from three to seven months. Forty-one percent of the patients experienced more than 50 percent improvement in their migraine condition. However, adverse effects were common and consisted of polymenorrhea (86 percent), breakthrough bleedings (64 percent), depression (18 percent), and amenorrhea (14 percent).

Menopausal Estrogen Therapy

The estrogens used most frequently for menopausal therapy are the conjugated estrogens obtained from the urine of pregnant mares (Premarin, UK/US) or synthetic estradiol (Progynova, UK; Estrace, US). The usual dose of Premarin is 0.6 mg, and that of estradiol is 1 mg per day. The medications are often given cyclically in combination with a progestogen to prevent endometrial hyperplasia. However, this is not necessary; the estrogen can be given daily with a small dose of progestogen or the progestogen can be given cyclically.

Like migraine patients on oral contraceptives, patients on menopausal estrogen therapy have attacks more frequently. In a study, 49 percent of a group of 147 patients had more than 4 attacks per month, as compared to 27 percent of 92 women who were not on hormonal treatment.[11] In the group of 78 patients on menopausal estrogen therapy, 58 percent improved after decycling the estrogen therapy and decreasing the dose by at least one-half. Improvement again was defined as a decrease in frequency of the attacks by at least 60 percent.

Stress

Stress is a very common rather than potent trigger factor. In a recent *population* study, 44 percent of the 119 identified migraine patients indicated stress as a trigger factor.[13] Of the same patients, 20 percent indicated alcohol as a trigger factor, 11 percent pointed to weather changes, and 10 percent named dietary products. In a *prospective* study of 49 patients who recorded 121 attacks during a period of two months, 54 percent of the attacks coincided with emotional stress.[14] However, the attacks triggered by stress typically do not occur during the stressful event but afterward. This was evident in a *prospective* study of five patients who recorded their headaches and 5 mood variables 2 times per day for 38 to 61 days.[15] The mood variables recorded and rated were nervousness, angriness, alertness, happiness, and ability to concentrate. Only headache and alertness showed cyclical trends, whereas the other mood variables fluctuated around the zero line (Figure 6.4). The cycles of headache and alertness were out of phase with each other by one or two days, with increased alertness *before* and decreased alertness *during* the migraine attack. The increased alertness before the migraine attack could be an indication of increased stress during that time.

In another *prospective* study, 17 patients recorded their headaches and 10 mood variables 3 times per day for 21 to 75 days.[16] The mood variables were all found to be low during headache and the day before. However, energy and ease were particularly and consistently low on the day before, especially when followed by severe headache. This indicates that the patients felt particularly tired and constrained on the day *before* a severe headache.

112 *Management of Migraine*

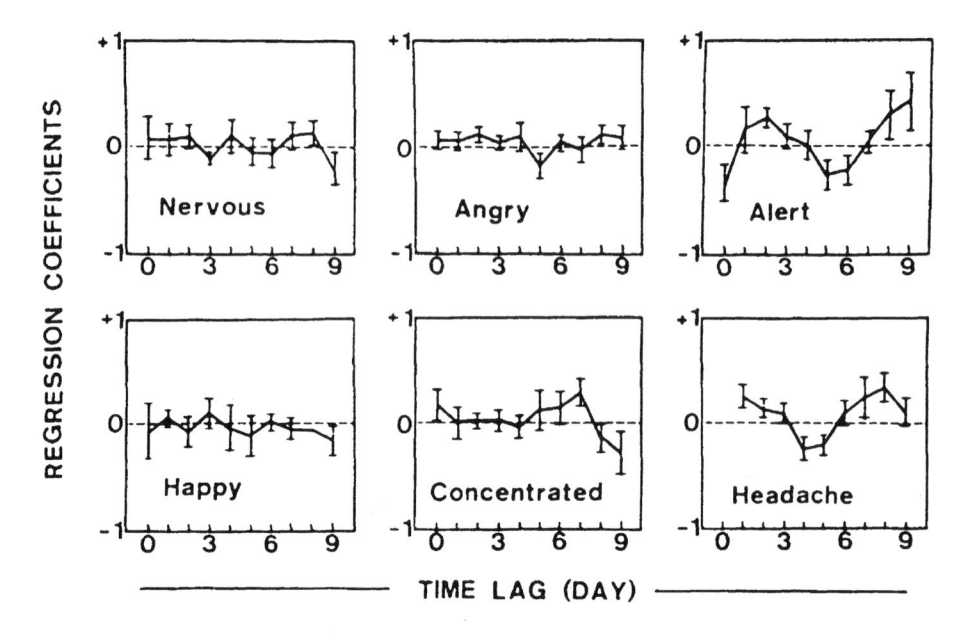

FIGURE 6.4 Mean regression coefficients as functions of the time lag (in days) between measurement of the independent (mood) variables and the dependent variable (headache) for a group of five migraine patients. From Dalkvist J, Ekbom K, Waldenlind E. Headache and mood: A time-series analysis of self-ratings. Cephalalgia 1984; 4:45–52 with permission.

In a *prospective* study of 19 patients, the changes in mood and daily hassles were determined during the 24 hours preceding the occurrence of migraine headache.[17] When the headache came about in the evening or during the night, the occurrence of daily hassles (i.e., stress) was increased during the preceding afternoon. When the headache came about in the morning, there was increased fatigue at 8 AM and the occurrence of daily hassles was increased the day before. When the headache came about in the afternoon, there was increased tenseness at 6 PM of the preceding day and increased alertness at 11 PM. On the day of the headache, the stressfulness of the daily hassles was increased at 8 AM and there was increased tenseness, irritability, and annoyance at 1 PM before the onset of the headache.

Weather Changes

In a *prospective* study, 44 patients recorded the dates of their attacks over periods of six months.[18] In total, 960 attacks were recorded, and the occurrence of these attacks was plotted against daily records of barometric pressure. The highest number of attacks was recorded on Fridays and Saturdays (i.e., at the end of the work week), and the lowest was on Mondays and Tuesdays. The frequency of the attacks was the highest between September and November, and the lowest in February and March. The mean barometric pressure on days during which attacks occurred was significantly higher than on days during which no attacks occurred. The frequency of attacks was also significantly lower when the barometric pressure at 6 AM was lower than 1005 millibar. An increase in barometric pressure of more than 15 millibar during the preceding 24 hours was also associated with a significant decrease in the frequency of attacks.

In a *questionnaire* study of 138 migraine patients, 30 percent indicated exposure to sun as a trigger factor of their attacks.[19] Exposure to sun is directly related to barometric pressure, as higher pressures are associated with clearer weather and, therefore, with more exposure to sun. However, migraine patients are also more sensitive to light in general both during *and* between the attacks (Figure 6.5).[20]

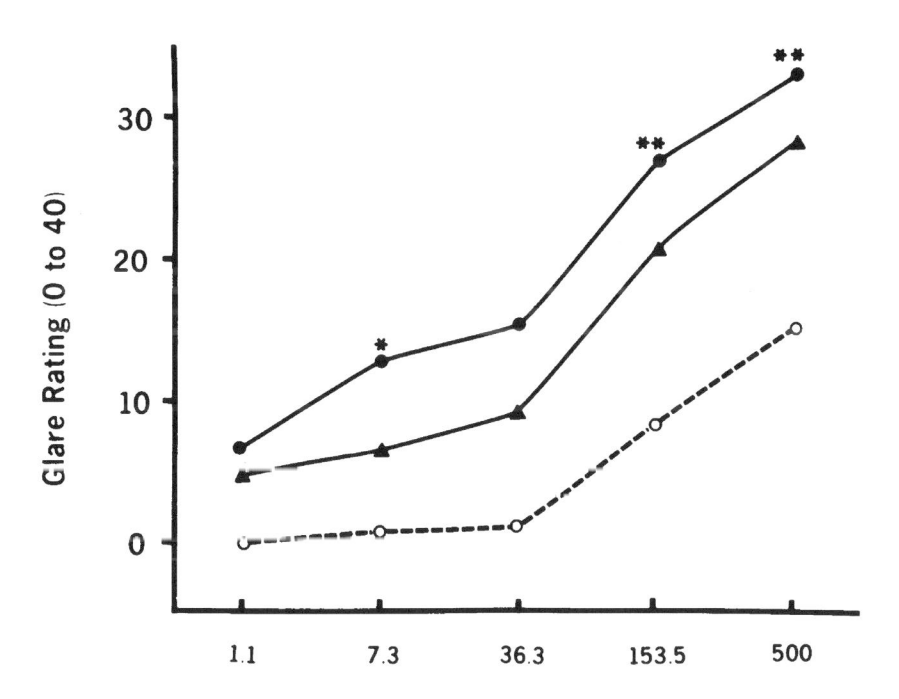

FIGURE 6.5 Glare ratings in migraine patients during (n = 21; closed circles) and between attacks (n = 18; triangles) as compared to controls (n = 20; open circles). From Drummond PD. A quantitative assessment of photophobia in migraine and tension headache. Headache 1986; 26:465–469 with permission.

Dietary Products

In a survey of almost 500 migraine patients, 19 percent indicated chocolate as a definite trigger factor, 18 percent named cheese, and 11 percent pointed to citrus fruits.[21] In addition, 29 percent indicated alcohol as a definite trigger factor. In another survey of 429 migraine patients, 16 percent reported precipitation of headache by cheese or chocolate, and nearly always by both.[22] With regard to alcohol, 18 percent of the patients indicated sensitivity to *all* alcoholic drinks, while 12 percent were sensitive to red wine but not to white wine. Twenty-eight percent pointed to beer as a trigger factor of headache. There was a significant correlation between sensitivity to cheese and chocolate on the one hand and red wine and beer on the other. However, there was no correlation between sensitivity to diet in general and to alcohol in general.

In a *questionnaire* study, 1,883 women with migraine recorded for three months all foods and drinks consumed in the 24 hours preceding the attack.[23] A total of 2,313 recorded attacks showed consumption of cheese in 40 percent, chocolate in 33 percent, alcohol in 23 percent, and citrus fruits in 21 percent. Fasting (i.e., going without food for five hours during the day or thirteen hours during the night) preceded 67 percent of the attacks. However, only 14 percent of the attacks were attributed to foods or drinks consumed in the preceding 24 hours, and (remarkably) only 2 percent were attributed to fasting. In a study of 12 migraine patients, 6 developed an attack after fasting for 19 hours.[24] However, the effect of fasting probably is not mediated by hypoglycemia. In a study of 20 migraine patients, the induction of moderately severe hypoglycemia (mean blood sugar level of 20 mg/100 ml) by injection of insulin brought on attacks in only two.[25]

Chocolate as a trigger factor of migraine was studied in a double-blind, placebo-controlled, *parallel* trial.[26] The trial involved 20 patients, all of whom completed the study. The dose of the chocolate was 40 gram. The patients were followed for 32 hours. In the chocolate group, 42 percent of the patients developed an attack, as opposed to none in the placebo group. The median time of onset of the attack was 22 hours with a range of 3.5 to 27 hours. Chocolate contains large quantities of a biogenic amine, *beta-phenylethylamine.* This amine is a directly-acting sympathomimetic that stimulates the postsynaptic alpha-adrenergic receptors.[27] It constricts the extracranial arteries and an attack possibly occurs when this effect wears off and rebound vasodilation occurs.

When cheese is allowed to mature, it contains large quantities of another biogenic amine, *tyramine.* This is an indirectly acting sympathomimetic that releases catecholamines from the sympathetic nerve terminals. It also constricts the extracranial arteries and may cause an attack by the same mechanism as that indicated above for beta-phenylethylamine. Tyramine was studied in a double-blind, placebo-controlled, *crossover* trial.[28] The trial involved 80 patients, all of whom completed the study. The dose of tyramine was 200 mg. The patients were followed for 24 hours. Twenty-five percent of the patients developed a headache after tyramine, compared to 29 percent after placebo.

Citrus fruits contain yet another biogenic amine, *octopamine.* This amine acts as a false neurotransmitter, replacing the catecholamines from the sympathetic nerve terminals.

Food additives can also act as trigger factors, though no studies are available. The food additives that have been implicated are *sodium nitrite, monosodium glutamate,* and *aspartame.* Sodium nitrite is often added to meat to preserve its red color. It is present in such cured-meat products as frankfurter, bacon, salami, and ham. Monosodium glutamate is a food additive used extensively in the preparation of some Chinese dishes. Aspartame is an artificial sweetener that is 150 to 200 times sweeter than sugar and is present in diet foods.

In a *questionnaire* study of 113 patients, 11 percent indicated aspartame as a definite trigger factor.[29] Sodium nitrite is a vasodilator that causes flushing of the face within 30 minutes. The vasodilation caused by the additive activates the sympathetic nervous system resulting in vasoconstriction. The headache possibly develops when the sympathetic nervous system activity decreases and rebound vasodilation occurs. The delay in the occurrence of the attack is explained by this indirect mechanism by which sodium nitrite and other vasodilators, like alcohol, may bring on an attack. Monosodium glutamate also was shown recently to act as a vasoconstrictor, and its vasoconstrictor effect was potentiated by tyramine.[30]

Caffeine is the last dietary ingredient and vasoconstrictor reviewed here. It is present in particular in coffee (50 to 100 mg per 8 oz), tea (25 to 50 mg per 8 oz), and cola drinks (15 to 25 mg per 12 oz). Caffeine brings about an attack on withdrawal from the body. Caffeine withdrawal often occurs during weekends, partially because of oversleeping, delaying the first cup of coffee.

In a *questionnaire* study of 101 patients, 30 percent experienced attacks on weekends.[31] These patients consumed more than two times as much caffeine per day than those without weekend migraine. The mean caffeine consumption of the patients was 734 mg per day with a surprising range from 510 to 1,253 mg. The patients with weekend migraine also woke up later on Saturdays and Sundays. They slept an average of 1.8 hours longer with a range of a half to three hours. Waking up with headache also was studied in 4 patients during 29 nights in the sleep laboratory.[32] In these patients, the occurrence of headache on awakening or the development of headache within one hour after getting up was associated with an increased sum total of sleep stages III, IV and REM. In a *retrospective* study of 494 migraine patients, oversleeping was mentioned by 24 percent as a trigger factor of headache and lack of sleep by 31 percent.[33]

References

1. Johannes CB, Linet MS, Stewart WF, et al. Relationship of headache to phase of the menstrual cycle among young women: A daily diary study. Neurology 1995; 45:1076–1082.
2. Epstein MT, Hockaday JM, Hockaday TDR. Migraine and reproductive hormones throughout the menstrual cycle. Lancet 1975; 1:543–548.
3. Chen TC, Leviton A. Headache recurrence in pregnant women with migraine. Headache 1994; 34:107–110.
4. Somerville BW. The role of estradiol withdrawal in the etiology of menstrual migraine. Neurology 1972; 22:355–365.
5. Somerville BW. The role of progesterone in menstrual migraine. Neurology 1971; 21:853–859.
6. Magos AL, Zilkha KJ, Studd JWW. Treatment of menstrual migraine by oestradiol implants. J Neurol Neurosurg Psychiatry 1983; 46:1044–1046.
7. De Lignieres B, Vincens M, Mauvais-Jarvis P, et al. Prevention of menstrual migraine by percutaneous oestradiol. Br Med J 1986; 293:1540.
8. Smits MG, Van der Meer YG, Pfeil JPJM, et al. Premenstrual migraine: Effect of Estraderm TTS and the value of contingent negative variation and exteroceptive temporalis muscle suppression test. Headache 1993; 34:103–106.
9. Ryan RE. A controlled study of the effect of oral contraceptives on migraine. Headache 1978; 17:250–252.
10. Dalton K. Migraine and oral contraceptives. Headache 1976; 15:247–251.
11. Kudrow L. The relationship of headache frequency to hormone use in migraine. Headache 1975; 15:36–40.
12. Somerville BW, Carey HM. The use of continuous progestogen contraception in the treatment of migraine. Med J Aust 1970; 1:1043–1045.
13. Rasmussen BK. Migraine and tension-type headache in a general population: Precipitating factors, female hormones, sleep pattern and relation to lifestyle. Pain 1993; 53:65–72.
14. Henryk-Gutt R, Rees WL. Psychological aspects of migraine. J Psychosom Res 1973; 17:141–153.
15. Dalkvist J, Ekbom K, Waldenlind E. Headache and mood: A time-series analysis of self-ratings. Cephalalgia 1984; 4:45–52.
16. Harrigan JA, Kues JR, Ricks DF, Smith R. Moods that predict coming migraine headaches. Pain 1984; 20:385–396.
17. Spierings ELH, Sorbi MJ, Maassen GH. Psychological precedents of migraine in relation to the time of onset of the attack. In preparation.
18. Cull RE. Barometric pressure and other factors in migraine. Headache 1981; 21:102–104.
19. Vijayan N, Gould S, Watson C. Exposure to sun and precipitation of migraine. Headache 1980; 20:42–43.
20. Drummond PD. A quantitative assessment of photophobia in migraine and tension headache. Headache 1986; 26:465–469.
21. Peatfield RC, Glover V, Littlewood JT, et al. The prevalence of diet-induced migraine. Cephalalgia 1984; 4:179–183.

22. Peatfield RC. Relationships between food, wine, and beer-precipitated migrainous headaches. Headache 1995; 35:355–357.
23. Dalton K. Food intake prior to migraine attack—Study of 2,313 spontaneous attacks. Headache 1975; 15:188–193.
24. Blau JN, Cumings JN. Method of precipitating and preventing some migraine attacks. Br Med J 1966; 2:1242–1243.
25. Pearce J. Insulin-induced hypoglycemia in migraine. J Neurol Neurosurg Psychiatry 1971; 34:154–156.
26. Gibb CM, Davies PTG, Glover V, et al. Chocolate is a migraine-provoking agent. Cephalalgia 1991; 11:93–95.
27. Gonsalves A, Johnson ES. Possible mechanism of action of beta-phenylethylamine in migraine. J Pharm Pharmacol 1977; 29:646.
28. Ziegler DK, Stewart R. Failure of tyramine to induce migraine. Neurology 1977; 27:725–726.
29. Lipton RB, Newman LC, Cohen JS, Solomon S. Aspartame as a dietary trigger of headache. Headache 1989; 29:90–92.
30. Merritt JE, Williams PB. Vasospasm contributes to monosodium glutamate-induced headache. Headache 1990; 30:575–580.
31. Couturier EGM, Hering R, Steiner TJ. Weekend attacks in migraine patients: Caused by caffeine withdrawal? Cephalalgia 1992; 12:99–100.
32. Dexter JD. The relationship between stages III + IV + REM sleep and arousals with migraine. Headache 1979; 19:364–369.
33. Robbins L. Precipitation factors in migraine: A retrospective review of 494 patients. Headache 1994; 34:214–216.

CHAPTER 7

Headache and Migraine in Childhood

Migraine in children is by far not as common as it is in adults, but it is still very prevalent. A review of population studies revealed a prevalence of migraine of 3.4 percent in boys and 4.0 percent in girls.[1] The prevalence increases sharply as the children enter their teens, a time at which the gender gap also widens.

In a cohort study of 2,921 children in Finland, the prevalence of migraine was 2.7 percent at the age of seven and 10.6 percent at age 14.[2] At the age of 7, 2.9 percent of the boys and 2.5 percent of the girls were affected, but the numbers increased to 6.4 and 14.8 percent respectively at age 14. As the children grew older, also considerable changes occurred in their migraine attacks. In particular, the headaches more often became unilateral, less often associated with nausea or vomiting and more often preceded by a visual aura (Table 7.1). The family history remained about the same and was positive in 81 percent at the age of 7 and in 73 percent at 14 (average: 75 percent).

Of the children who had migraine at the age of 7, 22 percent no longer had attacks at age 14. In 37 percent, the attacks had become milder at age 14 and in 41 percent were unchanged or more severe. The boys did somewhat better than the girls; 63 percent of them improved compared with 53 percent of the girls. With regard to the age of onset, of the children who had migraine

TABLE 7.1
Features of the migraine attack at age seven and fourteen

	Age seven	*Age fourteen*
Visual aura	19 percent	38 percent
Unilateral headache	44 percent	71 percent
Nausea/vomiting	81 percent	40 percent

From Sillanpaa M, 1983 with permission.[2]

120 *Management of Migraine*

at age 14, 35 percent of the boys and 22 percent of the girls experienced their first attack *before* school age.

Migraine in childhood was followed into adulthood in a cohort study of 9,059 children in Sweden.[3] In this study, the prevalence of migraine increased from 2.5 to 5.3 percent from the age of 7 to age 15. Of the 146 children in the study who had migraine, the 73 with "more pronounced" migraine were followed until they were 30 years or older (Figure 7.1). On the average, these 73 children had experienced their first attack at age 6. As teenagers or young adults, 38 percent of them still experienced attacks, whereas 62 percent of them had been free of attacks for at least 2 years. At the age of 30 or older, 60 percent still experienced attacks and only 40 percent had been free of attacks for at least 2 years. Of the 73 adults, 47 had children and 32 percent of them had one child with migraine. These 15 children represented 17 percent of the 90 children born to the adults.

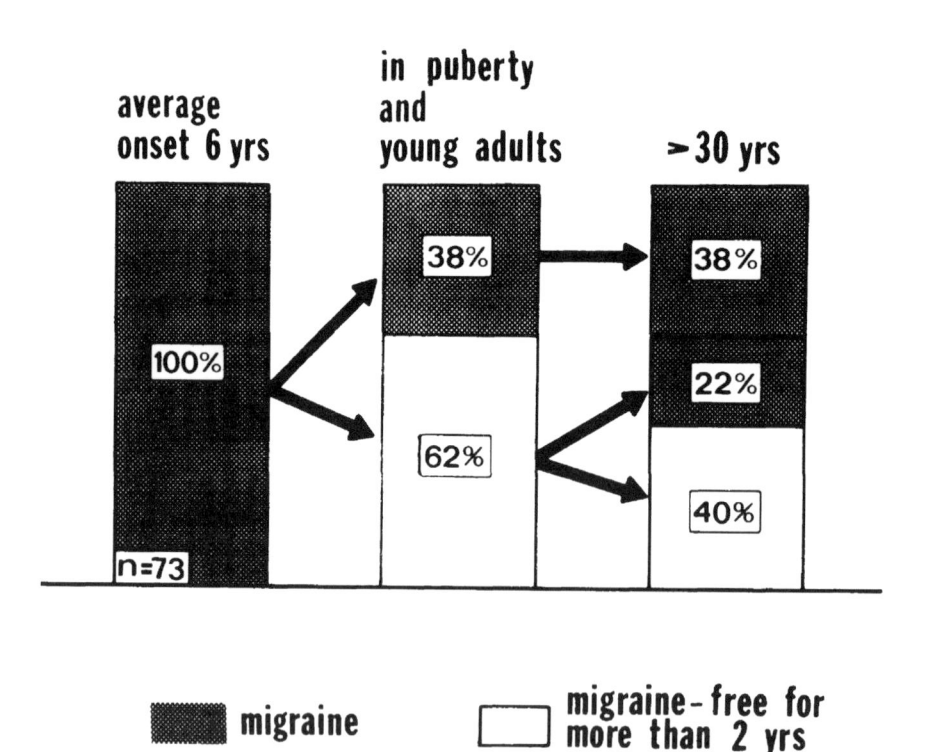

FIGURE 7.1 Follow-up of 73 children with "more pronounced" migraine from school age through puberty into adulthood. From Bille B. Migraine in childhood and its prognosis. Cephalalgia 1981; 1:71–75 with permission.

Migraine

Migraine attacks in children are generally shorter in duration but more frequent in occurrence than in adults. In a study of 300 children with migraine, 61 percent experienced headaches that were shorter than 5 hours.[4] In 80 percent of the children, the headaches lasted shorter than 10 hours, and only 4 percent experienced headaches longer than 24 hours. With regard to the frequency of the headaches, in 57 percent they occurred once or twice per month and in 39 percent once per week or more. The onset of the headaches is generally during the day and rarely do the headaches wake the child out of sleep at night. In the study, 17 percent of the children experienced headaches on awakening in the morning and in only 4 percent did the headaches wake the child at night.

Migraine headaches in children are also more commonly located bilaterally than in adults. Of the children in the study, 65 percent experienced headaches located across the forehead, 31 percent in one temple or the other, and 4 percent in both temples. The headaches generally are also associated with nausea or vomiting, which was the case in 100 percent of the children in the study. Thirteen percent of the children experienced a visual aura in the form of stars, flashes, spots, circles, or loss of vision. Eleven percent experienced blurring of vision, 5 percent reported double vision, and 2 percent spoke of micropsia. The attacks were brought on by traveling in 9 percent, by cold weather in 8 percent, by excessive exercise in 4 percent, by watching television in 3 percent, by bright sunlight in 2 percent, and by certain foods in 2 percent. On ophthalmological examination, 7 percent of the children required glasses, but none obtained relief from their attacks after receiving the glasses! However, children with migraine may benefit from wearing *red-(FL41)-tinted glasses*, especially at school, to filter out the shortwave-length flicker, produced by fluorescent lights. This was determined in a placebo-controlled, *parallel* study in which the placebo consisted of blue- as opposed to red-tinted glasses.[5] The glasses were worn by the children for at least eight hours per day. The trial involved 20 children between 8 and 14 years old, 16 of whom completed the study. The treatment periods were four months in duration, preceded by a baseline period of four weeks. The frequency of the attacks decreased by 74 percent from baseline in the red-tinted group and *increased* by 22 percent in the blue-tinted group. The intensity and duration of the attacks did not change significantly from baseline in either group. Adverse effects or cosmetic objections did not occur. Actually, *all* children experienced a reduction in light sensitivity between the migraine attacks, which made them happy.

With regard to *traveling* as a trigger factor in childhood migraine, 45 percent of children with migraine are susceptible to motion sickness.[6] This was determined in a study of 60 children between the ages of 5 and 20. The incidence of motion sickness in a comparable group of 60 children with epilepsy was 7 percent. The same study found that children with migraine walk in their sleep more often.[7] This was the case in 30 percent of the children with migraine as opposed to 7 percent of the children with epilepsy.

Stress as a trigger factor was studied in 37 migraine-afflicted children who were mostly between 8 and 14 years old.[8] Of these children, 86 percent indicated stress as a trigger factor of their attacks. In comparison, light was indicated as a trigger factor by 56 percent, hunger by 35 percent, lack of sleep by 35 percent, foods by 24 percent, cold environment by 18 percent, and fatigue by 11 percent. On psychological examination, 17 percent of the children were found to suffer from anxiety and 11 percent from depression. In a population study of adults with migraine, the prevalence of anxiety and *major* depression was determined as 10 and 15 percent respectively.[9] The comparable figures for the group of controls were 2 and 7 percent, respectively.

Differential Diagnosis

Headache caused by brain tumor is an important differential diagnosis of migraine in childhood. Brain tumors represent the second most common group of cancers in childhood after the leukemias. They generally are highly invasive and progress rapidly. A *retrospective* study of 105 children with brain tumors revealed that 69 percent of them experienced headaches.[10] The children were between 1 and 16 years old, but 64 percent of them were younger than 11. The headaches were generalized in location in 50 percent, occipital in 28 percent, and unilateral in 22 percent. They were associated with vomiting in 78 percent, which was daily in 11 percent and intractable in 3 percent. The headaches were particularly severe or prolonged in 13 percent and changed over time in frequency, intensity, or time of occurrence in 31 percent. They were present on awakening in the morning or woke the child out of sleep at night in a surprisingly high 67 percent. Of the children with headache caused by a brain tumor, 55 percent had an abnormal physical examination within two weeks of onset of the headache, 85 percent within two months, and *all* within six months. The physical examination included a neurological *and* ophthalmological examination. The latter consisted of examination of the pupils, fundi, visual fields, extraocular movements, *and* visual acuity.

Abortive Migraine Treatment

For the abortive treatment of migraine in childhood, the simple analgesics are generally adequate. However, aspirin is better avoided in children under the age of 12 because of the risk of Reye's syndrome. Over that age, children can be treated with the adult dose of the medication, that is, 1,000 mg followed twice if necessary by 500 mg with intervals of a half hour. The dose of acetaminophen in children under the age of 12 is one-quarter to one-half of the adult dose, that is, 250 to 500 mg followed twice if necessary by half of the initial dose with intervals of a half hour. The dose of ibuprofen in children under the age of 12 is also a quarter to a half of the adult dose, that is, 100 to 200 mg repeated twice if necessary with intervals of a half hour.

For use in children, both acetaminophen and ibuprofen are available in suspensions. However, prior to treatment with an analgesic, children always should be given an antiemetic first. The reasons for this are twofold: First, migraine attacks in children almost always are associated with gastrointestinal symptoms, and second, children with migraine often respond with relief of their headache to treatment with an antiemetic.

The antiemetics that can be used in children are the gastrokinetic and antihistamine antiemetics. The gastrokinetic antiemetics are domperidone (Motilium, UK; not available in the US) and metoclopramide (Maxolon or Primperan, UK; Reglan, US). For use in children, domperidone is available as a suspension in a concentration of 5 mg per 5 ml. In children under the age of 12, the dose of the medication is 5 to 10 mg. Metoclopramide is also available as a suspension in a concentration of 5 mg per 5 ml. The dose of the medication in children under the age of 12 is 2.5 to 5 mg.

The antihistamine antiemetics are diphenhydramine (Benadryl, UK/US) and promethazine (Phenergan, UK/US). For use in children, diphenhydramine is available as a suspension in a concentration of 7 (UK) or 12.5 mg (US) per 5 ml. In children under the age of 12, the dose of the medication is 12.5 to 25 mg. Promethazine is also available as a suspension in a concentration of 5 (UK), 6.25 or 25 mg (US) per 5 ml. The dose of the medication in children under the age of 12 is 10 to 25 mg. Over that age, children can be given the adult dosages of the medications.

The antiemetics mentioned do not have contraindications. Domperidone generally does not cause adverse effects, whereas metoclopramide can cause restlessness and, occasionally, dystonia. Diphenhydramine and promethazine generally cause drowsiness. However, the drowsiness is not necessarily an adverse effect, as it often allows the child to sleep, thereby facilitating the recovery from the headache.

Preventive Migraine Treatment

The medications studied in the preventive treatment of childhood migraine are propranolol, clonidine, pizotifen, trazodone, flunarizine, and nimodipine. A summary of the reported efficacies of propranolol, trazodone, and nimodipine are presented in Table 7.2.

Propranolol

Propranolol (Inderal, UK/US) was studied in a double-blind, placebo-controlled, *crossover* trial.[11] The trial involved 32 children between the ages of 7 and 16, 28 of whom completed the study. The dose of the medication was 20

TABLE 7.2
Reported efficacies of propranolol, trazodone, and nimodipine in the preventive treatment of migraine in children

Medication	Efficacy	Study
Propranolol 60–120 mg/day	70 percent decrease in attack frequency from pretrial condition	Ludvigsson, 1974[11]
Trazodone 1 mg/kg/day	43–45 percent decrease in attack frequency from baseline	Battistella, et al., 1993[15]
Nimodipine 30–60 mg/day	15–30 percent decrease in attack frequency from baseline	Battistella, et al., 1990[17]

mg 3 times per day in children weighing less than 35 kg and 40 mg 3 times per day in children weighing 35 kg or more. The treatment periods were 12 weeks in duration, preceded by a dose-adjustment period of 1 week. In comparison to the pretrial condition, the frequency of the attacks decreased by 70 percent during treatment with propranolol and by 9 percent during placebo treatment. With regard to adverse effects, 7 percent of the children experienced mild insomnia during treatment with propranolol.

Clonidine

Clonidine (Catapres, UK/US) was studied in two double-blind, placebo-controlled trials. The first trial used a *parallel* design and involved 57 children below the age of 15, all of whom completed the study.[12] The dose of the medication was 0.025 mg 2 times per day in children weighing 40 kg or less and 0.025 mg 3 times per day in children weighing more than 40 kg. The treatment periods were two months in duration. In comparison to the pretrial condition, the number of headaches decreased by 17 percent in the clonidine group and by 30 percent in the placebo group. The number of *severe* headaches decreased by 85 percent in the clonidine group and by 79 percent in the placebo group. Adverse effects were experienced by 39 percent of the children in the clonidine group and by 21 percent in the placebo group. The most common adverse effects experienced by the children in the clonidine group were fatigue and nausea.

The second was a *crossover* trial and involved 51 children between the ages of 7 and 14, 43 of whom completed the study.[13] The dose of the medication was 0.025 mg once daily during the first month, two times per day during the second month and three times per day during the third month. The treatment periods were three months in duration. The frequency and duration of the attacks did not differ significantly between the two treatments. No adverse effects were observed during treatment with clonidine.

Pizotifen

Pizotifen (Sanomigran, UK; not available in the US) was studied in a double-blind, placebo-controlled, *crossover* trial.[14] The trial involved 47 children between the ages of 7 and 14, 39 of whom completed the study. The dose of the medication was 0.5 mg two times per day for the first six weeks and three times per day for the second six weeks. The treatment periods were three months in duration. The frequency and duration of the attacks did not differ significantly between the two treatments. Adverse effects were experienced by 10 percent of the children during treatment with pizotifen and by 8 percent during placebo treatment.

Trazodone

Trazodone (Molipaxin, UK; Desyrel, US) was studied in a double-blind, placebo-controlled, *crossover* trial.[15] The trial involved 40 children between the ages of 7 and 18, 35 of whom completed the study. The dose of the medication was 1 mg/kg per day in three divided doses. The treatment periods were 12 weeks in duration, preceded by a baseline period of 4 weeks. The frequency of the attacks decreased in the first treatment period by 45 percent from baseline during treatment with trazodone and by 49 percent during placebo treatment (Figure 7.2). However, during the second treatment period, the frequency of the attacks decreased by 43 percent during treatment with trazadone and *in*creased by 56 percent during placebo treatment. The duration of the attacks showed similar changes during the first and second treatment periods. Adverse effects did not occur with the medication, in particular no drowsiness or changes in school performance were observed.

Flunarizine

Flunarizine (Sibelium; not available in the UK or US) was studied in a double-blind, placebo-controlled, *crossover* trial.[16] The trial involved 70 children between the ages of 5 and 11, 63 of whom completed the study. The dose of the medication was 5 mg once daily at bedtime. The treatment periods were 12 weeks in duration, preceded by a baseline period of 4 weeks. The

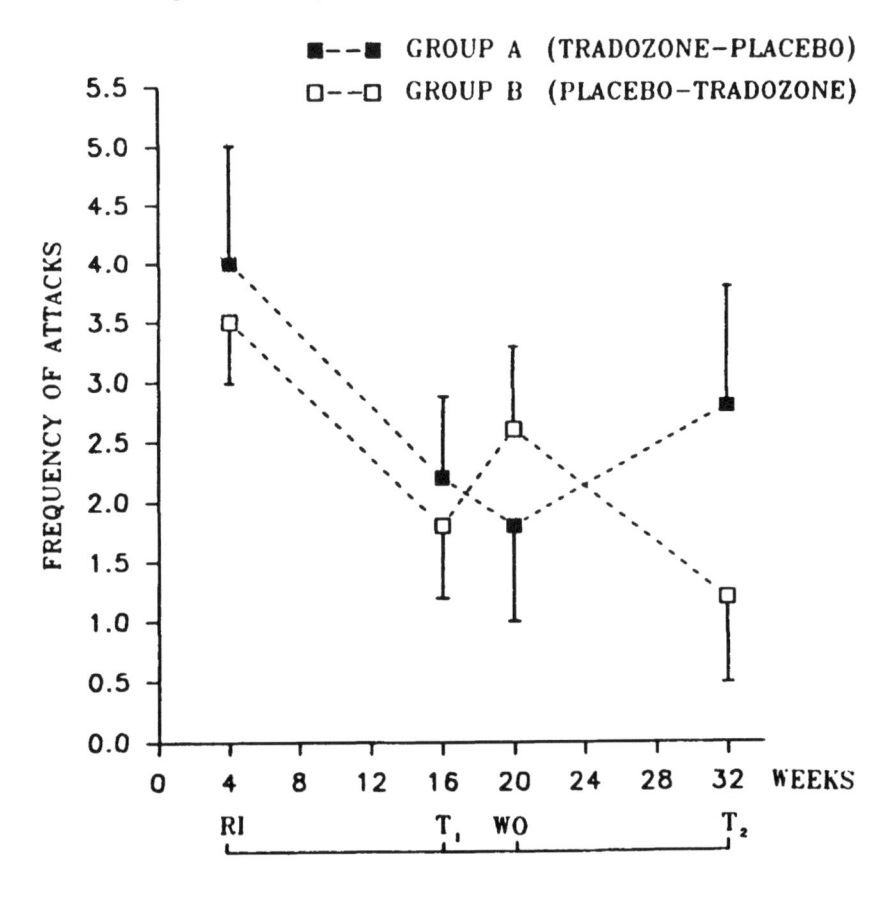

FIGURE 7.2 Frequency of migraine attacks during treatment with trazodone, 1 mg/kg per day, and placebo in 35 children with migraine. From Battistella PA, Ruffilli R, Cernetti R, et al. A placebo-controlled crossover trial using trazodone in pediatric migraine. Headache 1993; 33:36–39 with permission.

frequency and duration of the attacks decreased significantly from baseline during treatment with flunarizine but not during treatment with placebo. With regard to adverse effects, 10 percent of the children experienced drowsiness during treatment with flunarizine and 22 percent experienced weight gain.

Nimodipine

Nimodipine (Nimotop, UK/US) was studied in a double-blind, placebo-controlled, *crossover* trial.[17] The trial involved 37 patients between the ages of 7 and 18, 30 of whom completed the study. The dose of the medication was 10

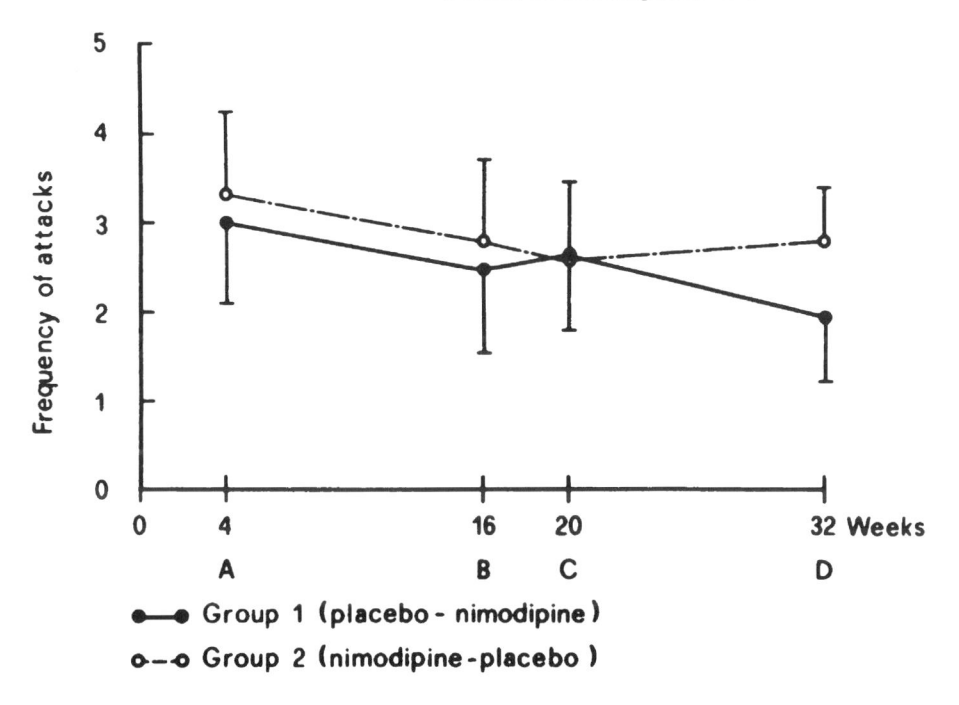

FIGURE 7.3 Frequency of migraine attacks during treatment with nimodipine, 10 to 20 mg three times per day, and placebo in 30 children with migraine. From Battistella PA, Ruffilli R, Moro R, et al. A placebo-controlled crossover trial of nimodipine in pediatric migraine. Headache 1990; 30:264–268 with permission.

mg 3 times per day in children weighing less than 40 kg, 16 mg 3 times per day in children weighing between 40 and 50 kg, and 20 mg 3 times per day in children weighing more than 50 kg. The treatment periods were 12 weeks in duration, preceded by a baseline period of 4 weeks. The frequency of the attacks decreased in the first treatment period by 15 percent from baseline during treatment with nimodipine and by 17 percent during placebo treatment (Figure 7.3). However, during the second treatment period, the frequency of the attacks decreased by 30 percent during treatment with nimodipine and increased by 8 percent during placebo treatment. The duration of the attacks decreased significantly and to the same extent during both treatment periods.

Efficacy

Clonidine and pizotifen were found to be ineffective, and nimodipine was only modestly effective, which leaves propranolol, trazodone, and flunarizine. Rounded estimates of the efficacy of these medications are 70 percent for propranolol, 60 percent for flunarizine, and 45 percent for trazodone. Of the medications, trazodone seems to have the least adverse effects, followed by propranolol and flunarizine. Propranolol is, however, probably the first choice, because of its higher efficiency, followed by flunarizine and trazodone.

The dose of propranolol is 60 to 120 mg per day and has to be given in two divided doses, but it can be given once daily when the long-acting preparation is used. Contraindications for the use of propranolol are sinus bradycardia and obstructive pulmonary disease, including asthma. In addition, it should be used with great care in children with diabetes mellitus or depression. Its most common adverse effects are lethargy, fatigue, depression, and insomnia.

The dose of flunarizine is 5 mg once daily, preferably taken at bedtime. The medication causes mild drowsiness and sometimes weight gain or depression. The dose of trazodone is 1 mg/kg per day. The medication is available in the United Kingdom as a liquid and in the United States as a dividose tablet. The dose has to be given in two to four divided doses because of the short half-life of the medication. The most common adverse effects of trazodone are drowsiness, dry mouth, and lightheadedness. There are no contraindications to the use of either flunarizine or trazodone.

References

1. Goldstein M, Chen TC. The epidemiology of disabling headache. Adv Neurol 1982; 33:377–390.
2. Sillanpaa M. Changes in the prevalence of migraine and other headaches during the first seven school years. Headache 1983; 23:15–19.
3. Bille B. Migraine in childhood and its prognosis. Cephalalgia 1981; 1:71–75.
4. Congdon PJ, Forsythe WI. Migraine in childhood: A study of 300 children. Dev Med Child Neurol 1979; 21:209–216.
5. Good PA, Taylor RH, Mortimer MJ. The use of tinted glasses in childhood migraine. Headache 1991; 31:533–536.
6. Barabas G, Matthews WS, Ferrari M. Childhood migraine and motion sickness. Pediatrics 1983; 72:188–190.
7. Barabas G, Ferrari M, Matthews WS. Childhood migraine and somnambulism. Neurology 1983; 33:948–949.
8. Maratos J, Wilkinson M. Migraine in children: A medical and psychiatric study. Cephalalgia 1982; 2:179–187.
9. Merikangas KR, Angst J, Isler H. Migraine and psychopathology. Results of the Zurich Cohort Study of Young Adults. Arch Gen Psychiatry 1990; 47:849–853.
10. Honig PJ, Charney EB. Children with brain tumor headaches. Am J Dis Child 1982; 136:121–124.
11. Ludvigsson J. Propranolol used in prophylaxis of migraine in children. Acta Neurol Scand 1974; 50:109–115.

12. Sillanpaa M. Clonidine prophylaxis of childhood migraine and other vascular headache. A double blind study of 57 children. Headache 1977;17:28–31.
13. Sills M, Congdon P, Forsythe I. Clonidine and childhood migraine: A pilot and double-blind study. Dev Med Child Neurol 1982; 24:837–841.
14. Gillies D, Sills M, Forsythe I. Pizotifen (Sanomigran) in childhood migraine. A double-blind controlled trial. Eur Neurol 1986; 25:32–35.
15. Battistella PA, Ruffilli R, Cernetti R, et al. A placebo-controlled crossover trial using trazodone in pediatric migraine. Headache 1993; 33:36–39.
16. Sorge F, De Simone R, Marano E, et al. Flunarizine in prophylaxis of childhood migraine. A double-blind, placebo-controlled, crossover study. Cephalalgia 1988; 8:1–6.
17. Battistella PA, Ruffilli R, Moro R, et al. A placebo-controlled crossover trial of nimodipine in pediatric migraine. Headache 1990; 30:264–268.

CHAPTER 8

Cluster Headache and Paroxysmal Hemicrania

Cluster Headache

Cluster headache is a vascular headache condition that is related to migraine in certain aspects of its pathogenesis. Consequently, it responds to some of the same medications. However, it differs from migraine in other aspects of its pathogenesis and in many aspects of its clinical presentation. Cluster headache is not nearly as common as migraine and, according to a population study, affects less than one out of 1,000 people.[1] As opposed to migraine, it mostly affects men, with a male to female ratio of at least 10 to 1. The age of onset of cluster headache is usually between 20 and 40, which is much later than migraine. The clinical presentation of cluster headache is very consistent; therefore, the condition generally is relatively easy to diagnose.

The clinical presentation of cluster headache is characterized by the daily (or almost daily) occurrence of headaches. The intensity of the headache is generally severe to very severe. They last from a half to two hours and occur on the average once or twice per day. The headaches have a preference for occurring during the night, waking the patient in the early hours of the night. In so-called *episodic* cluster headache, the headaches occur daily (or almost daily) for two to eight weeks. The episodes of headaches are separated by remissions which last 6 to 12 months. In so-called *chronic* cluster headache, the headaches occur daily (or almost daily) for at least a year without remission. Chronic cluster headache is divided further into primary and secondary, depending on whether the condition was initially episodic. In 85 percent of patients with cluster headache, the condition is episodic, and in 15 percent it is chronic (i.e., 10 percent primary and 5 percent secondary).

The headaches of cluster headache are *always* unilateral and in 90 percent of those afflicted, *always* affect the same side of the head (i.e., have a fixed laterality). They are usually located in the eye, sometimes also in the temple. In the eye, the pain is invariably sharp and steady and is often described as "a hot poker going through it." In the temple, the pain is usually throbbing, behaving in the same way it does in migraine. The headaches come about relatively rapidly and build up to their maximum intensity in five to ten minutes. They very often end as quickly as they come about.

The headaches generally are not associated with the systemic autonomic symptoms as seen in migraine. They generally are not associated with nausea or vomiting or with phonophobia; when photophobia occurs, it usually only affects the painful eye. The eye, however, very often shows autonomic symptoms of its own, such as reddening and tearing. Also, the upper eyelid may droop and may become edematously swollen. The ipsilateral nostril often shares the autonomic symptoms of the eye, becoming stuffy and running. In the temple, as in migraine, the frontal branch of the superficial temporal artery may become prominent.

The psychophysical make-up of patients with cluster headache has been described as the "leonine-mouse syndrome."[2] The syndrome refers to the husky appearance of many of the patients, exhibiting such leonine features in the face as ruddy complexion, deep furrows, and broad prominent

TABLE 8.1
Summary of the clinical features of cluster headache

Feature	Finding
Prevalence	0.07 percent
Age of onset	20–40 years
Gender distribution	90 percent men
Temporal pattern	
Episodic	85 percent
Chronic	
Primary	10 percent
Secondary	5 percent
Attacks	
Duration	1/2–2 hours
Frequency	1–2/day
Episodes	
Duration	2–8 weeks
Remissions	6–12 months
Laterality	
Right	50 percent
Left	40 percent
Either	10 percent
Local autonomic symptoms	
Ocular	85 percent
Nasal	70 percent

From Kudrow L, 1980 with permission.[3]

chin and eyebrows. In contrast to the outside appearance, however, the individual may be timid, with increased dependency needs—the mouse living inside the lion. Cluster headache patients generally also smoke and drink excessively, habits that have been related to the above-described physical appearance. During an actual attack, cluster headache patients often also behave like lions and pace up and down the floor. The clinical features of cluster headache are summarized in Table 8.1.[3]

Pathogenesis of Cluster Headache

Like migraine, the headache of cluster headache responds abortively to vasoconstrictor medications, such as ergotamine and sumatriptan (*vide infra*). Therefore, it is likely that extracranial arterial vasodilation is also an important mechanism in the pathogenesis of cluster headache. However, in contrast to migraine, the focus of the dilation is centered more in the eye than in the temple. Evidence for dilation of the intraocular arteries is provided by a study of the corneal indentation pulse amplitude.[4] The amplitude is increased on the side of the pain during attacks of cluster headache. In a recent magnetic resonance angiography study of a patient with cluster headache, dilation of the ipsilateral ophthalmic artery was actually observed during the attack (Figure 8.1).[5]

The mechanism of neurogenic inflammation probably also is involved in the pathogenesis of cluster headache. Evidence for this is provided by a study of the level of calcitonin gene-related peptide in blood collected from the external jugular vein.[6] Calcitonin gene-related peptide is a potent vasodilator involved in neurogenic inflammation and released from the primary sensory nerve endings. It was found to be increased during nitroglycerine-induced attacks of cluster headache with subsequent normalization after resolution of the pain (Figure 8.2).

The local autonomic symptoms (i.e., the reddening and tearing of the eye and the stuffiness and running of the ipsilateral nostril) can be explained by a *decrease* in sympathetic and *increase* in parasympathetic activity.[7] The local decrease in sympathetic activity not only explains the reddening of the eye but also the drooping of the upper eyelid and the narrowing of the pupil as is sometimes seen. The local increase in parasympathetic activity explains the tearing of the eye and stuffiness and running of the ipsilateral nostril and also may contribute to the narrowing of the pupil.

I have suggested that the local decrease in sympathetic and increase in parasympathetic activity reflects a shift in autonomic balance (Figure 8.3),[7] implicating the involvement of centers of autonomic regulation in the pathogenesis of cluster headache. These centers are located in the hypothalamus, which also harbors the centers that drive the biological rhythms to which cluster headache in its clinical presentation is very clearly subjected.

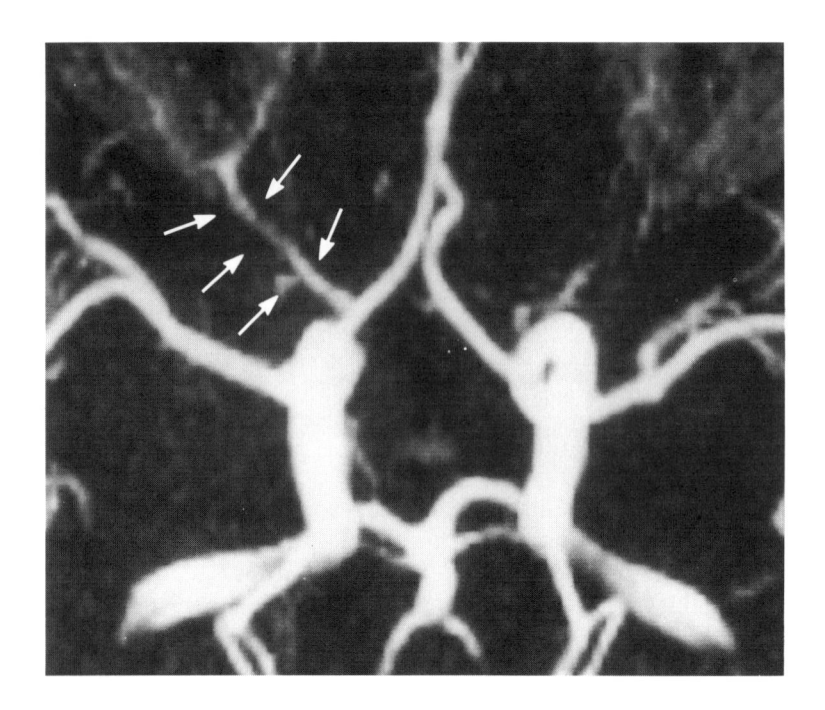

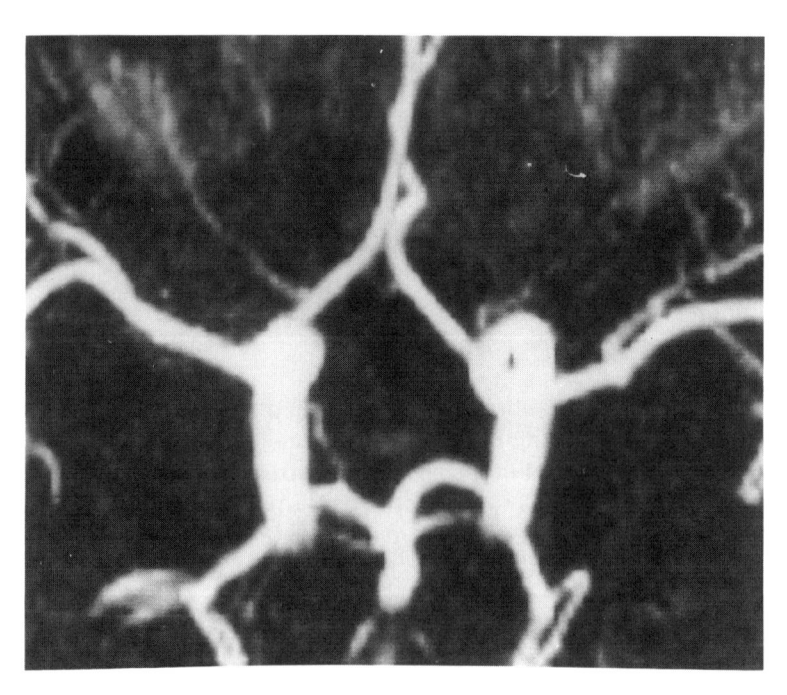

FIGURE 8.1 Magnetic resonance angiography (transaxial projections) during (top) and after an attack of cluster headache (bottom), showing dilation of the ipsilateral ophthalmic artery (arrows) during the attack. From Waldenlind E, Ekbom K, Torhall J. MR-angiography during spontaneous attacks of cluster headache: A case report. Headache 1993; 33:291–295 with permission.

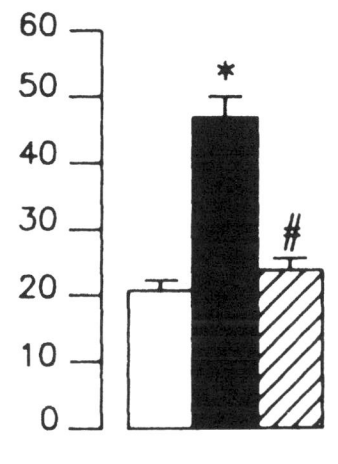

FIGURE 8.2 Levels of calcitonin gene-related peptide in blood drawn from the external jugular vein before (open column) and during nitroglycerine-induced attacks of cluster headache (black column) and afterwards (hatched column). From Fanciullacci M, Alessandri M, Figini M, et al. Increase in plasma calcitonin gene-related peptide from the extracranial circulation during nitroglycerine-induced cluster headache attacks. Pain 1995; 60:119–123 with permission.

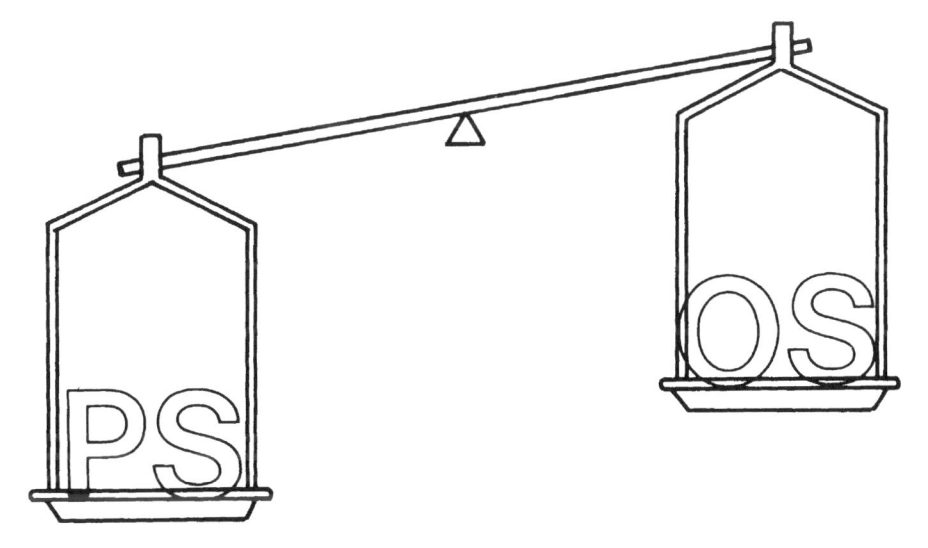

FIGURE 8.3 The local autonomic symptoms of cluster headache as a manifestation of a shift in local autonomic balance in favor of the parasympathetic (PS) and to the detriment of the (ortho)sympathetic nervous system activity (OS).

Treatment of Cluster Headache

The treatment of cluster headache, like that of migraine, consists of three parts: elimination of trigger factors and abortive and preventive treatment. However, the emphasis is on preventive treatment because of the high frequency of occurrence of the attacks. The elimination of trigger factors consists of instructing the patients *not* to drink alcohol and *not* to take naps while in an episode of headaches. Alcohol and daytime napping are the only two factors to which cluster headache consistently responds with the development of an attack. After the consumption of alcohol (or any other vasodilator), the headache takes from 30 to 45 minutes to develop, independent of the quantity of alcohol consumed.

In the abortive treatment of cluster headache, three specifically administered medications have the highest efficacy and are reviewed here. These medications are ergotamine by *sublingual tablet* (Lingraine, UK; Ergomar or Ergostat, US), sumatriptan by *subcutaneous injection* (Imigran, UK; Imitrex, US), and oxygen by *inhalation.* The medications that are effective in the preventive treatment of cluster headache are methysergide (Deseril, UK; Sansert US), verapamil (Cordilox, UK; Isoptin, US), prednisone, and lithium.

Ergotamine and sumatriptan are potent arterial vasoconstrictors. Therefore, they are contraindicated in patients with hypertension, coronary artery disease, or prominent risk factors for cardiovascular disease.

Ergotamine

Ergotamine is most effective when given as a sublingual tablet to promote rapid absorption. This preparation generally is tolerated well by patients with cluster headache, whereas it is *not* by patients with migraine. The ergotamine sublingual tablet was studied in an *open* trial of 50 patients.[8] The dose of the medication was 2 mg, repeated if necessary every 15 minutes with a maximum of 3. The patients treated 10 attacks with ergotamine. In 70 percent of the patients, the medication aborted at least 7 out of 10 attacks. The peak response occurred within 10 to 12 minutes after the initiation of treatment.

Sumatriptan

Sumatriptan was studied in a double-blind, placebo-controlled, *crossover* trial.[9] The trial involved 49 patients, 39 of whom completed the study. The dose of the medication was 6 mg given by subcutaneous injection. The efficacy of sumatriptan was 74 percent as compared to 26 percent with placebo. Efficacy was defined as a reduction in headache intensity from moderate, severe or very severe to mild or no headache within *15 minutes* of treatment (Figure 8.4). Adverse effects were experienced by 35 percent of the patients during treatment with sumatriptan and by 26 percent during placebo treatment. In an *open* study, 138 patients with cluster headache treated 6,353 attacks (mean 46) with subcutaneous sumatriptan over a period of three months.[10] Headache relief as defined above was obtained in a median of 96 percent of the attacks treated. There was no indication of decreased efficacy or increased frequency of the attacks with long-term treatment. Adverse effects occurred in 28 percent of the attacks treated with the medication. There was no increase in adverse effects with frequent use of the medication.

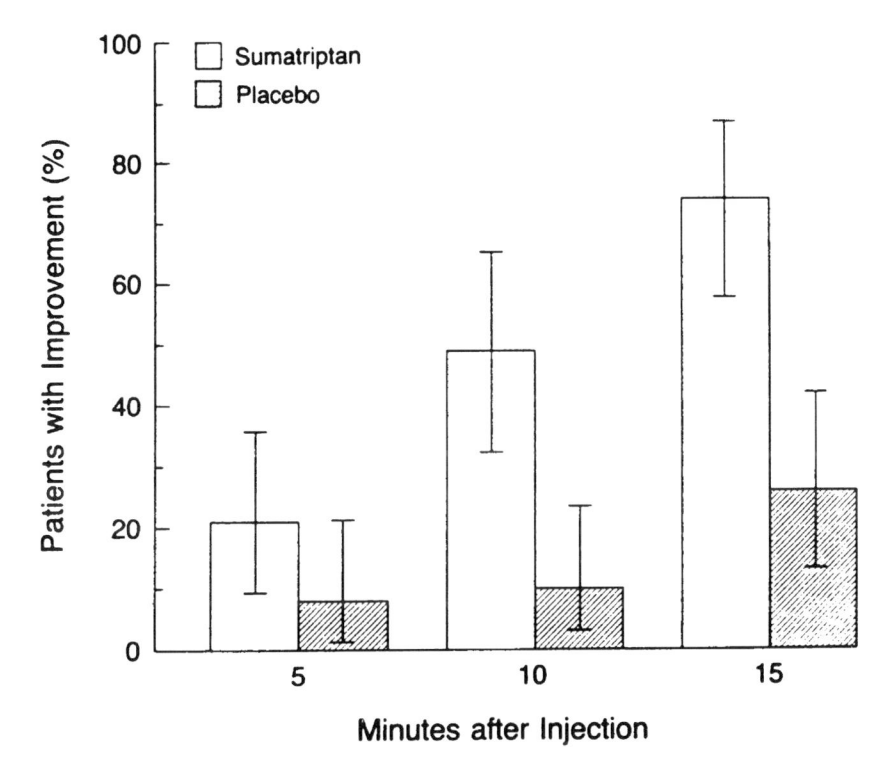

FIGURE 8.4 Efficacy of sumatriptan, 6 mg by subcutaneous injection, in the abortive treatment of cluster headache, defined as a reduction in headache intensity from moderate, severe or very severe to mild or no headache. From the Sumatriptan Cluster Headache Study Group, Treatment of acute cluster headache with sumatriptan. N Engl J Med 1991; 325:322–326 with permission.

Oxygen

Oxygen inhalation also was studied in a double-blind, placebo-controlled, *crossover* trial.[11] The trial involved 19 patients, 11 of whom completed the study (treating up to 6 attacks). The patients inhaled 100 percent oxygen for up to 15 minutes at the onset of the headache, at a rate of six liters per minute. The placebo consisted of inhalation of air. In 56 percent of the patients, inhalation of oxygen provided complete or substantial relief in 80 percent or more of the attacks, compared to 7 percent with air.

Oxygen inhalation also was studied in an *open* trial of 50 patients.[8] The patients inhaled 100 percent oxygen for 15 minutes at the onset of the headache, at a rate of 7 liters per minute. They treated 10 attacks with oxygen inhalation. In 82 percent of the patients, oxygen aborted at least 7 out of 10 attacks. The peak response occurred within four to six minutes after the initiation of treatment! Adverse effects did not occur.

138 Management of Migraine

Methysergide, prednisone, and lithium

With regard to preventive treatment, methysergide, prednisone, and lithium were studied in an *open* trial of 92 patients.[12] Of these patients, 77 had episodic and 15 chronic cluster headache. They were treated first for 21 days with methysergide, 8 mg per day in divided doses. Subsequently, they were treated with prednisone for 21 days, starting at 40 mg per day in divided doses, followed by a gradual taper. The patients with chronic cluster headache then were treated with lithium, 300 mg two times per day for one week, followed by 900 mg per day for an additional two weeks. Improvement was defined as a reduction in frequency or intensity of the headaches by 75 percent or more.

Treatment with *methysergide* resulted in improvement of 46 percent of the patients, 53 percent of those with episodic cluster headache, and 7 percent of those with chronic cluster headache. Treatment with *prednisone* resulted in improvement of 71 percent of the patients, 77 percent of those with episodic cluster headache, and 40 percent of those with chronic cluster headache. Treatment with *lithium* resulted in improvement of 87 percent of the patients with chronic cluster headache (Table 8.2).

Prednisone also was studied in a double-blind, placebo-controlled, *crossover* trial.[14] The trial involved 19 patients, all of whom completed the study. The dose of the medication was either 30 mg for abortive treatment *or* 20 mg every other day for preventive treatment. The abortive treatment provided relief in 89 percent of patients. The preventive treatment significantly reduced the frequency of the attacks, as compared to placebo treatment.

Verapamil

Verapamil was studied in an *open* trial which involved 48 patients, 45 of whom completed the study.[13] Thirty-three of the patients had episodic and 15 chronic cluster headache. The medication was used in a sustained-release (SR) preparation. The initial dose was 120 mg SR two times per day. The dose was increased if necessary until headache relief was obtained or adverse

TABLE 8.2
Efficacy of preventive treatment in cluster headache

Medication	Episodic cluster headache	Chronic cluster headache
Methysergide	53 percent	7 percent
Verapamil	73 percent	60 percent
Prednisone	77 percent	40 percent
Lithium	—	87 percent

Data obtained from Kudrow, 1978[12] and Gabai, Spierings, 1989.[13]

effects developed. Improvement was defined as a reduction in headache frequency of more than 75 percent.

Treatment with verapamil resulted in improvement of 69 percent of the 48 patients, (i.e., including the three patients who dropped out of the study). Of the patients with episodic cluster headache, 73 percent improved and of those with chronic cluster headache, 60 percent (Table 8.2). In the patients with episodic cluster headache, the relief was obtained with an average dose of 354 mg SR per day (range: 240 to 600 mg) within an average of 1.7 weeks (range: 1 to 6 weeks). In the patients with chronic cluster headache, the relief was obtained with an average dose of 572 mg SR per day (range: 120 to 1200 mg) within an average of 5 weeks (range: 1 to 20 weeks). The adverse effects were relatively mild and mostly consisted of constipation (12 percent) and drowsiness (6 percent).

Abortive treatment

With regard to *abortive* treatment, oxygen inhalation should be the mainstay. Oxygen inhalation is very effective and does not have adverse effects or contraindications. It should be used with an appropriate face mask to allow as close to 100 percent concentration as possible. The rate of inhalation is 8 to 10 liters per minute and it should be used for 10 to 15 minutes at the onset of the headache. The ergotamine sublingual tablet or sumatriptan injection can be used when the oxygen is not available or as a rescue. As mentioned, these medications are contraindicated in patients with hypertension, coronary artery disease, or prominent risk factors for cardiovascular disease. The dose of ergotamine is 2 mg, and that of sumatriptan is 6 mg. The medications can be used two times in 24 hours with an interval of minimally one hour. Ergotamine can cause nausea, vomiting, and leg cramps. Sumatriptan can cause flushing, numbness, and tightness, especially in the upper chest, anterior neck, and face.

Preventive treatment

With regard to *preventive* treatment, verapamil is the first choice in patients with episodic or chronic cluster headache. It is very effective in both conditions and generally is tolerated well. The medication can be given two times per day when the sustained-release (SR) preparation is used. The initial dose is 120 mg SR two times per day and is increased by 120 mg per week. When a dose of 480 mg per day is reached, an electrocardiogram and echocardiogram should be performed. The purpose of the electrocardiogram is to determine the atrioventricular conduction, and the echocardiogram can be used to rule out heart muscle disease. If both are unremarkable, the dose of the medication can be increased further if necessary. The electrocardiogram should be repeated within two or three days after every subsequent increase in dose. When peripheral edema occurs, a diuretic can be added. Verapamil is contraindicated in patients with sick sinus syndrome or atrioventricular block. Adverse effects are constipation and sometimes impotence or male infertility.

When verapamil is ineffective or not adequately effective, the second choice is lithium. This medication can be given instead of verapamil or can be added to it. The dose of lithium is 300 mg two times per day and if necessary can be increased with increments of 300 mg. The blood level should be determined regularly to ensure that it is *not* in the toxic range (i.e., above 1.5 mEq/liter). It is also advisable to determine the electrolyte levels and kidney function regularly, and once per year the thyroid function should be checked. Adverse effects of lithium are nausea, stomach upset, drowsiness, and tremor of the hands. Lithium does not have contraindications, but it should be used with care in patients with electrolyte imbalance or who need sodium restriction or diuretic therapy.

Prednisone is the preventive medication of choice when rapid relief is required. It usually is effective within the first one or two days of treatment. The medication can be initiated in a dose of 60 mg per day, maintained for three days. The dose is subsequently *de*creased by 5 mg every two days. At the same time that the prednisone is started, verapamil or lithium can be initiated for long-term preventive treatment. The dose of these medications can be gradually increased while the headaches are controlled by the prednisone. Adverse effects of the prednisone are indigestion, insomnia, fluid retention, and weight gain. The medication is contraindicated in patients with an infection, hypertension, peptic ulcer disease, diabetes mellitus, or diverticulosis.

Because methysergide is *not* effective in chronic cluster headache, it should be used only in patients with episodic cluster headache. In episodic cluster headache, it should be used during the cluster episodes only and discontinued during the remissions. When used in this way, the fibrotic adverse effects of the medication are generally not a concern. The dose of the medication is 1 or 2 mg four times per day. The medication is contraindicated in patients with hypertension, coronary artery disease, peripheral vascular disease, valvular heart disease, pulmonary disease, collagen vascular disease, or fibrotic conditions. Adverse effects are nausea, indigestion, and leg cramps.

Paroxysmal Hemicrania[15]

Paroxysmal hemicrania is a variant of cluster headache. It is very similar to cluster headache in its clinical presentation and may be confused easily with it. It differs from cluster headache in two clinical features, the duration and the frequency of the headaches. The duration of the headaches is much shorter, lasting between 10 and 30 minutes, compared to a half to two hours in cluster headache. The frequency of the headaches is also much higher, attacks occurring from 5 to 15 times per 24 hours, compared to once or twice per 24 hours in cluster headache. Like migraine but unlike cluster headache, the condition is two or three times more common in women than in men.

Paroxysmal hemicrania also differs from cluster headache in its treatment. It is a condition that responds with *complete* relief to preventive treatment with indomethacin (Indocid, UK; Indocin, US). The dose of indomethacin is 25 or 50 mg four times per day. The medication should be taken with the meals and at bedtime with food to protect the stomach. After some time, the dose very often can be decreased or the medication discontinued without recurrence of the headaches. The medication is contraindicated in patients with peptic ulcer disease, or bleeding disorder. When the patient does not tolerate the indomethacin, verapamil should be tried in the same regimen as it is used in cluster headache.

References

1. D'Alessandro R, Gamberini G, Benassi G, et al. Cluster headache in the Republic of San Marino. Cephalalgia 1986; 6:159–162.
2. Graham JR. Cluster headache. Headache 1972; 11:175–185.
3. Kudrow L. Cluster headache. New York: Oxford University Press, 1980.
4. Hørven I, Nornes H, Sjaastad O. Different corneal indentation pulse pattern in cluster headache and migraine. Neurology 1972; 22:92–98.
5. Waldenlind E, Ekbom K, Torhall J. MR-angiography during spontaneous attacks of cluster headache: A case report. Headache 1993; 33:291–295.
6. Fanciullacci M, Alessandri M, Figini M, et al. Increase in plasma calcitonin gene-related peptide from the extracranial circulation during nitroglycerine-induced cluster headache attacks. Pain 1995; 60:119–123.
7. Spierings ELH. The involvement of the autonomic nervous system in cluster headache. Headache 1980; 20:218–219.
8. Kudrow L. Response of cluster headache attacks to oxygen inhalation. Headache 1981; 12:1–4.
9. Sumatriptan Cluster Headache Study Group. Treatment of acute cluster headache with sumatriptan. N Engl J Med 1991; 325:322–326.
10. Ekbom K, Krabbe A, Micelli G, et al. Cluster headache attacks treated for up to three months with subcutaneous sumatriptan (6 mg). Cephalalgia 1995; 15:230–236.
11. Fogan L. Treatment of cluster headache. A double-blind comparison of oxygen vs air inhalation. Arch Neurol 1985; 42:362–363.
12. Kudrow L. Comparative results of prednisone, methysergide and lithium therapy in cluster headache. In: Greene R. Current Concepts in Migraine Research. New York: Raven Press, 1978:159–163.
13. Gabai IJ, Spierings ELH. Prophylactic treatment of cluster headache with verapamil. Headache 1989; 29:167–168.
14. James JL. The treatment of cluster headaches with prednisone. Dis Nerv Sys 1975; 36:375–376.
15. Spierings ELH. Episodic and chronic paroxysmal hemicrania. Clin J Pain 1992; 8:44–48.

Index

Abortive treatment, 27–29
   adverse effects, 53
   antiemetics, 27–28, 52, 123
   childhood migraine, 122–123
   cluster headache, 135–140
   duration of action, 53–55, 58
   efficacy, 51–52, 124
   narcotic analgesics, 28–29, 35–36
   nonsteroidal anti-inflammatory
      analgesics, 28, 31–35, 52, 53, 57, 140
   rebound cycle, 55
   simple analgesics, 28, 29–31, 52, 53, 57, 123
   summary, 59
   vasoconstrictor medications, 28, 29, 36–59, 133
Acetaminophen, 29
   childhood migraine, 123
   combination with isometheptene, 37, 57
   combination with codeine, 35
   combination with diazepam, 31
   combination with domperidone, 31
   combination with metoclopramide, 31
   comparison with aspirin, 30
   comparison with ibuprofen, 30–31
   dosage, 57, 59
Adalat, 66, 87 *See also* Nifedipine
Alcohol
   cluster headache, 135–136
   migraine, 111, 114
Amitriptyline
   combination with beta-blockers, 99
   combination with clonidine, 99
   comparison with flunarizine, 99
   comparison with fluvoxamine, 80
   comparison with propranolol, 80
   contraindications, 98
   dosage, 97–98

   efficacy, 95
   migraine prevention, 66, 78–80, 100
   mode of action, 100
Amyl nitrite, 12, 14
Anafranil, 80 *See also* Clomipramine
Analgesics
   adverse effects, 53
   efficacy, 52
   migraine abortion, 28–29
   nonsteroidal anti-inflammatory
      analgesics, 28, 31–35, 52, 53, 57, 95, 96
   simple analgesics, 29–31, 52, 53, 57, 123
Anaprox *See also* Naproxen sodium
   migraine abortion, 32, 34–35
   migraine prevention, 66, 81
Anthranilic acids, 32
Anticholinergic antiemetics, 28
Antidepressants, tricyclic *See* Tricyclic antidepressants
Antidopaminergic antiemetics, 28
Antiemetics, 27–28, 52, 123
Antihistaminergic antiemetics, 28, 123
Anti-inflammatory analgesics *See* Nonsteroidal anti-inflammatory analgesics
Anxiety, in migraine sufferers, 122
Arterial vasodilation, extracranial, 9–10, 12–13, 15–18
Aspartame, as trigger factor, 115
Aspirin
   combination with metoclopramide, 29, 30, 48–49
   comparison with acetaminophen, 30
   comparison with acetaminophen plus codeine, 35
   comparison with metoprolol
   comparison with propranolol, 81
   comparison with sumatriptan, 48–49

143

Aspirin (Cont.):
childhood migraine, 122–123
dosage, 57, 59
duration of action, 54
efficacy, 95
migraine abortion, 29, 30, 35, 53, 122–123
migraine prevention, 66, 80–81, 95, 100
Atarax, 28 See also Hydroxyzine
Atenolol
comparison with propranolol, 73
contraindications, 97
dosage, 97
efficacy, 75, 95
migraine prevention, 66, 70, 73–74, 100
mode of action, 101
Aura symptoms See Migraine aura
Autonomic symptoms
cluster headache, 133, 135
migraine, 7

Barometric pressure, migraine, 112–113
Basilar migraine, 3, 5
Beer, as trigger factor, 114
Bellergal, 66–68, 96, 100
Benadryl, 28, 123 See also Diphenhydramine
Beta-receptor blockers
adverse effects, 96, 97
in combination, 99, 100
contraindications, 98
efficacy, 71–74, 95
migraine prevention, 70–78
mode of action, 100, 101
Betaloc, 66, 73 See also Metoprolol
Betaphenylethylamine, as trigger factor, 114
Betim, 66, 78 See also Timolol
Blocadren, 66, 78 See also Timolol
Blurring of vision, 8, 121
Brain tumor, childhood migraine differentiated from, 122
Butorphanol, 35–36, 52, 53

Cafergot
comparison with sumatriptan, 69
dosage, 59, 60
duration of action, 54–55
efficacy, 52
migraine abortion, 39–41, 49–50
Caffeine
combination with ergotamine, 37, 39–41, 49–50, 52, 55, 57–58
migraine abortion, 29, 34
as trigger factor, 115

Calcitonin gene-related peptide, 11–12, 133, 135
Calcium-entry blockers
adverse effects, 96, 98
contraindications, 98
dosage, 98
efficacy, 84, 95
migraine prevention, 84–89
mode of action, 100
Cardene, 66, 85 See also Nicardipine
Catapres See also Clonidine
childhood migraine, 123–127
migraine prevention, 66, 89
Cerebral blood flow
cluster headache, 132, 133
migraine, 9–10, 12–13, 15–18, 114–115
Cheese, as trigger factor, 114–115
Children, headache and migraine in, 119–127
Chlorpromazine, 28
Chocolate, as trigger factor, 114
Chronic daily headache, 22, 23–24
Chronic tension-type headache, 23–24
Citrus fruits, as trigger factor, 114, 115
Classic migraine, 1, 3
cerebral blood flow, 13–18
drug treatment, 55–57
pathogenesis, 13–18
symptoms, 8
Clomipramine, 80
Clonidine
adverse effects, 96, 98, 124, 125
childhood migraine, 123–127
combination with amitriptyline, 99
combination with pizotifen, 99
comparison with metoprolol, 91–92
comparison with propranolol, 91
contraindications, 98
dosage, 98
efficacy, 89, 95
migraine prevention, 66, 89, 91, 100, 123–127
mode of action, 101
Cluster headache, 2, 22, 131–133
pathogenesis, 133–135
treatment, 135–140
Codeine, 35, 52, 53
combination with acetaminophen, 35
comparison with aspirin, 35
Common migraine, 1, 3, 15–18
Compazine, 28, 43 See also Prochlorperazine
Complicated migraine, 3, 4, 25
Contraceptives, oral See Oral contraceptives
Cordilox, 66, 87, 136 See also Verapamil

Corgard, 66, 76 *See also* Nadolol
Cyclizine, 34
Cyproheptadine
  contraindications, 98
  dosage, 97
  migraine prevention, 66, 68–69, 100
  mode of action, 100

Decongestants, 37
Demerol, 43–44 *See also* Meperidine
Depakote, 66, 92 *See also* Valproate
Depression, in migraine sufferers, 122
Deseril, 66–68, 125, 136 *See also* Methysergide
DHE 45, 41 *See also* Dihydroergotamine
Diazepam, 31
Dichloralphenazone, 37, 60
Diclofenac, 31–33
Diet, as trigger factor, 111, 114–115, 121, 122
Digitolingual syndrome, 8, 9
Dihydergot, 41, 66 *See also* Dihydroergotamine
Dihydroergotamine
  adverse effects, 53, 58
  combination with metoclopramide, 43–45
  combination with prochlorperazine, 43
  comparison with meperidine plus promethazine, 43
  contraindications, 57–58
  dosage, 58, 59, 60, 96
  duration of action, 58
  efficacy, 52
  migraine prevention, 9, 66, 67, 96
  migraine abortion, 37, 41–46, 57
Diphenhydramine, 28, 123
Domperidone
  childhood migraine, 123
  combination with acetaminophen, 31
  dosage, 59
  migraine abortion, 27, 28, 31, 52, 53, 55, 57
Double vision, 121
Drug treatment *See* Abortive treatment; Preventive treatment

Elavil, 66, 78 *See also* Amitriptyline
Emotional stress, as trigger factor, 111–112
Enkephalin, 12, 13
Epilepsy, differentiating from migraine, 21
Epilim, 66, 92 *See also* Valproate
Episodic tension-type headache, 23–24
Ergomar, 136 *See also* Ergotamine
Ergostat, 136 *See also* Ergotamine

Ergot alkaloids
  adverse effects, 95
  efficacy, 67, 95
  migraine prevention, 66–68, 95, 96
  mode of action, 100
Ergotamine
  adverse effects, 53, 58, 139
  combination with caffeine, 34, 37, 40–41, 49–50, 52, 55, 57–58
  combination with cyclizine, 34
  combination with metoclopramide, 41
  combinatin with phenobarbital, 66
  comparison with Midrin
  comparison with naproxen sodium, 34
  comparison with tolfenamic acid, 35
  cluster headache, 133, 136, 139
  contraindications, 57–58, 139
  dosage, 58–59
  duration of action, 54–55, 58
  efficacy, 95
  migraine abortion, 9, 11, 34, 35, 37–41
  migraine prevention, 66–67, 95, 100
  withdrawal, 55
Estrace, 107, 111 *See also* Estradiol
Estraderm, 107 *See also* Estradiol
Estradiol, 107, 108, 110
Estrogen, migraine and, 107, 108–110
Estrogen cycle as trigger factor, 2, 105–110
Estrogen therapy, as trigger factor, 111
Ethinyl estradiol, 110
Exercise, as trigger factor, 121
Exposure to sun, as trigger factor, 113, 121
Extracranial arterial vasodilation, 9–10, 12–13, 15–18

Familial hemiplegic migraine *See* Hemiplegic migraine
Fasting, as trigger factor, 114
Faverin, 80 *See also* Fluvoxamine
Fenoprofen, 66, 80, 83
Flunarizine
  adverse effects, 96, 98, 125, 127
  childhood migraine, 123, 125, 127
  combination with pizotifen, 99
  comparison with metoprolol, 86
  comparison with nifedipine, 87–87
  comparison with pizotifen, 84–86
  comparison with propranolol, 86
  contraindications, 98, 127
  dosage, 98, 127
  efficacy, 84, 95, 127
  migraine prevention, 66, 83, 84–85, 87, 100, 123, 125, 127

Fluorescent lights, as trigger factor, 121
Fluoxetine, 80
Fluvoxamine, 80
  comparison with amitriptyline, 80
Follicle stimulating hormone, migraine and, 107, 108
Food additives, as trigger factor, 115
Foods, as trigger factors, 111, 114–115, 121, 122
Fortification spectra *See* Scintillating scotoma

Gastrointestinal symptoms, 52
  childhood migraine, 119, 121, 123
  drug treatment, 27–28
  migraine, 7, 8, 23
Gastrokinetic antiemetics, 28, 52, 123
Gynergen, 37, 39 *See also* Ergotamine

Headache
  brain tumor, 122
  causes, 21–25
  in childhood, 119–127
  chronic daily headache, 22, 23–24
  cluster headache, 2, 22, 131–140
  intracranial hemorrhage, 22
  meningitis, 21
  paroxysmal hemicrania, 2, 140
  tension-type vascular headache, 23–24
  vascular headache, 2–3, 22–24, 131–140
Hemicrania, paroxysmal *See* Paroxysmal hemicrania
Hemiplegic migraine, familial, 3, 4–5, 8
Hydroxyzine, 28
Hyperemia, 13–14
Hypoglycemia, as trigger factor, 114

Ibuprofen
  comparison with acetaminophen, 30–31
  childhood migraine, 123
  dosage, 57, 59
  migraine abortion, 29, 30–31, 123
IHS *See* International Headache Society
Imigran, 136 *See also* Sumatriptan
Imitrex, 45, 136 *See also* Sumatriptan
Inderal, 66, 70, 123 *See also* Propranolol
Indocid, 32, 34, 83, 140 *See also* Indomethacin
Indocin, 32, 34, 83, 140 *See also* Indomethacin

Indomethacin
  contraindications, 140
  dosage, 57, 59
  migraine abortion, 32, 34, 57
  migraine prevention, 84
  paroxysmal hemicrania, 140
Inflammation, migraine and, 10–11, 37, 100
International Headache Society (IHS), classification system, 3–4, 22
Intracranial hemorrhage, differentiating from migraine, 22
Ischemic stroke, 25
Isolated migraine aura, 1, 21
Isometheptene *See also* Midrin
  adverse effects, 53
  dosage, 59
  efficacy, 52
  migraine abortion, 37, 57
Isoptin, 66, 87, 136 *See also* Verapamil

Lack of sleep, as trigger factor, 115, 122
Light, as trigger factor, 122
Lingraine, 136 *See also* Ergotamine
Lithium, cluster headache, 136–140
Lopressor, 66, 73 *See also* Metoprolol
Luteinizing hormone, migraine and, 107, 108

Major depression, in migraine sufferers, 122
Maxolon, 27, 28, 123 *See also* Metoclopramide
Medihaler-Ergotamine, 41
Meningitis, differentiating from migraine, 21
Menopause, migraine incidence after, 106, 111
Menstrual cycle, as trigger factor, 2, 105–110
Meperidine, 43–44
  combination with promethazine, 44
  comparison with dihydroergotamine, 43
Methysergide
  adverse effects, 95, 96–97, 99, 140
  cluster headache, 136, 137–138, 140
  comparison with pizotifen, 69–70
  comparison with propranolol, 71–72
  in combination, 100
  contraindications, 140
  dosage, 96, 99
  efficacy, 68, 95
  migraine prevention, 66–68, 69–70, 100

Metoclopramide
  combination with aspirin, 29, 30, 48–49
  combination with dihydroergotamine, 43–45
  combination with ergotamine, 41
  combination with tolfenamic acid, 35
  migraine abortion, 27, 28, 31, 52, 53, 55
  use in childhood migraine, 123
Metoprolol
  comparison with aspirin, 81
  comparison with clonidine, 91–92
  comparison with flunarizine, 85
  comparison with pizotifen, 76
  comparison with propranolol, 74–76
  contraindications, 97
  dosage, 97
  efficacy, 72, 95
  migraine prevention, 66, 70, 73–76, 100
  mode of action, 101
Midrin *See also* Isometheptene
  adverse effects, 53
  comparison with ergotamine, 37
  dosage, 59
  efficacy, 52
  migraine abortion, 37, 57
Migraine *See also* Migraine aura; Migraine headache; Trigger factors
  brain tumor, differentiating from, 122
  cause, 15–18
  cerebral blood flow, 9–10, 13, 15–18, 114–115
  in childhood, 119–127
  chronic daily headache, differentiating from, 23–24
  classification, 3–4
  diagnosis, 4–5, 21–25, 122
  duration, 22
  epidemiology, ix, 119–120
  epilepsy, differentiating from, 21
  estrogen cycle and, 2, 105–110
  estrogen therapy and, 111
  foods and, 111, 114–115, 121, 122
  frequency, 2
  heredity, 1
  location of headache, 7, 23, 121
  meningitis, differentiating from, 21
  menopause and, 111
  menstrual migraine, 105–110
  oral contraceptives and, 110
  pathogenesis, 9–18, 114
  pregnancy and, 106, 107
  preventive treatment, 65–101, 123–127
  seeking medical treatment, ix–x
  stress and, 105, 111–112, 122

  subarachnoid hemorrhage, differentiating from, 22
  symptomatology, 7–9
  time of onset, 55
  transient ischemic attacks, differentiating from, 21
  treatment with drugs, x, 27–60, 122–123
  weather changes and, 111, 112–113, 121
Migraine aura, 1
  cause, 15–18, 25
  in children, 119, 121
  description, 8–9
  drug treatment, 27
  migraine with aura, 4
  pathogenesis, 12–18
Migraine aura without headache, 1, 3, 4, 21
Migraine complicated by stroke, 3, 4
Migraine process, 18
Migraine status, 3, 5, 22
Migraine with acute onset aura, 3, 4
Migraine with aura
  cerebral blood flow, 13–18
  diagnosis, 4
  drug treatment, 55–57
  estrogen cycle, 105
  pathogenesis, 13–18
  symptoms, 8
Migraine without aura, 1, 3, 4
  cerebral vasoconstriction, 15–18
  estrogen cycle, 105
  pathogenesis, 15–18
Migraine with prolonged aura, 3, 4
Migrainous infarction, 3, 4, 8, 9
Migwell, 34 *See also* Ergotamine
Molipaxin, 125 *See also* trazodone
Monosodium glutamate, as trigger factor, 115
Mood, as trigger factor, 111–112
Motilium, 27, 28, 123 *See also* Domperidone
Motion sickness, and migraine, 121–122

Nadolol
  comparison with propranolol, 77–78
  dosage, 97
  efficacy, 74, 95
  migraine prevention, 66, 70, 76–79, 100
  mode of action, 101
Nalfon, 66, 83 *See also* Fenoprofen
Naproxen, 53
Naproxen sodium
  comparison with ergotamine, 34
  comparison with pizotifen, 82–83
  comparison with propranolol, 81–82

148 Index

Naproxen sodium (*Cont.*):
  dosage, 57, 59
  efficacy, 95
  migraine prevention, 66, 80, 81–83, 95, 100
  migraine abortion, 32, 34–35
Naps, cluster headache, 135–136
Narcotic analgesics, 28–29, 35–36
National Institute of Neurological Diseases and Blindness (NINDB), classification system, 3
Nausea
  childhood migraine, 119, 121
  migraine, 4, 7, 28
  treatment, 27–28, 52, 123
Neurogenic inflammation
  cluster headache, 133
  migraine, 10–11, 37, 100
Neurokinin A, 11
Nicardipine, 66, 83, 85
Nifedipine
  adverse effects, 96
  comparison with flunarizine, 87–88
  comparison with pizotifen, 88
  comparison with propranolol, 88
  efficacy, 95
  migraine prevention, 66, 83, 87–87, 89, 100
Nimodipine
  adverse effects, 98
  childhood migraine, 123–127
  contraindications, 98
  dosage, 98
  efficacy, 95, 124
  migraine prevention, 66, 83, 87, 100, 123–127
  mode of action, 100
Nimotop, 66, 87, 125 *See also* Nimodipine
NINDB *See* National Institute of Neurological Diseases and Blindness
Nonsteroidal anti-inflammatory analgesics
  adverse effects, 53, 95
  contraindications, 57
  dosage, 57
  efficacy, 52, 95
  migraine abortion, 28, 31–35
  migraine prevention, 80–83, 95, 96
  paroxysmal hemicrania, 140
Numbness, 8

Octopamine, as trigger factor, 115
Odorphobia, 7, 23
Oligemia, 14, 16

Ophthalmoplegic migraine, 3, 5
Oral contraceptives, as trigger factor, 110
Oversleeping, as trigger factor, 115
Ovral, 110 *See also* Ethinyl estradiol
Oxygen inhalation, cluster headache, 136–137, 139

Paracetamol, 29 *See also* Acetaminophen
Parasympathetic activity, cluster headache, 133
Paroxysmal hemicrania, 2, 140
Periactin, 66, 68–69 *See also* Cyproheptadine
Pethidine, 43 *See also* Meperidine
Pharmacological treatment *See* Abortive treatment; Preventive treatment
Phenergan, 28, 123 *See also* Promethazine
Phenobarbital, with ergotamine, 66
Phenylephrine, 37
Phenylethylamine, as trigger factor, 114
Phenylpropanolamine, 37
Phonophobia, 7–8, 23
Photophobia
  childhood migraine, 121
  cluster headache, 132
  migraine, 7–8, 23, 113, 121
Pizotifen
  childhood migraine, 123, 125–127
  combination with flunarizine, 99
  comparison with beta-receptor blockers, 99
  comparison with clonidine, 99
  comparison with flunarizine, 84, 85
  comparison with methysergide, 69–70
  comparison with metoprolol, 76
  compariosn with naproxen sodium, 82–83
  comparison with nimodipine, 87
  contraindications, 98
  dosage, 97–98
  efficacy, 69, 95
  migraine prevention, 66, 68, 69–70, 100, 123, 125–127
  mode of action, 100
Prednisone
  adverse effects, 140
  cluster headache, 136, 137–138, 139–140
  contraindications, 140
Pregnancy, migraine incidence during, 106, 107
Premarin, 111
Preventive treatment, 65–101, 123–127
  beta-receptor blockers, 70–78, 95–101
  calcium-entry blockers, 83–89, 95, 96, 98, 100

childhood migraine, 123–127
cluster headache, 135–140
efficacy, 93–96
ergot alkaloids, 66–68, 95, 96, 100
estradiol, 107, 108–110
long-term, 97–100
menstrual migraine, 107, 109–110
nonsteroidal anti-inflammatory
    medications, 80–83, 95, 96
serotonin antagonists, 68–70, 95, 100
short-term, 95, 96–97, 100
tricyclic antidepressants, 78–80, 95
Primperan, 27, 28, 123 See also
    Metoclopramide
Procardia, 66, 87 See also Nifedipine
Prochlorperazine, 28, 43
Progesic, 66, 83 See also Fenoprofen
Progesterone, migraine and, 107, 108, 110
Progynova, 107, 111 See also Estradiol
Promethazine, 28, 44, 123
    combination with meperidine, 44
Propranolol
    adverse effects, 96, 124, 127
    childhood migraine, 123–124, 127
    comparison with amitriptyline, 80
    comparison with aspirin, 81
    comparison with atenolol, 73
    comparison with clonidine, 91
    comparison with flunarizine, 85
    comparison with metoprolol, 74–76
    comparison with methysergide, 71–72
    comparison with nadolol, 77–78
    comparison with naproxen sodium, 81–82
    comparison with nifedipine, 88
    comparison with timolol, 78
    contraindications, 127
    dosage, 97, 127
    efficacy, 71, 95, 124, 127
    migraine prevention, 66, 70–71, 97, 100, 123–124, 127
    mode of action, 101
Prozac, 80 See also Fluoxetine

Rebound cycle, 55
Red-tinted glasses, 121
Red wine, as trigger factor, 114
Reglan, 27, 123
Reticular activating system, 8, 18
Retinal migraine, 3, 5

Sanomigran, 66, 69, 125 See also Pizotifen
Sansert, 66–68, 136 See also Methysergide

Scintillating scotoma, 8, 9
Sensitivity See Odorphobia; Phonophobia; Photophobia
Sensory symptoms, 7–8, 23, 113
    migraine diagnosis, 21
    treatment, 27
Serotonin, 100
Serotonin antagonists
    efficacy, 69, 95
    migraine prevention, 68–70
    mode of action, 100
Serotoninergic vasoconstrictors, 36, 37–59
    contraindications, 57–58
Sibelium, 66, 84, 85, 125 See also
    Flunarizine
Simple analgesics
    adverse effects, 53
    childhood migraine, 123
    contraindications, 57
    dosage, 57
    efficacy, 52
    migraine abortion, 28, 29–31, 123
Sleep
    cluster headache, 135–136
    migraine, 115, 122
Sodium nitrite, as trigger factor, 115
Spreading depression, 12–13
Stadol, 35 See also Butorphanol
Status migrainosus, 3, 5, 22
Stemetil, 28, 43 See also Prochlorperazine
Stress, as trigger factor, 105, 111–112, 122
Subarachnoid hemorrhage, differentiating from migraine, 22
Substance P, 11
Sumatriptan
    adverse effects, 53, 139
    cluster headache, 133, 136, 137, 139
    comparison with aspirin plus metoclopramide, 48–49
    comparison with Cafergot, 49
    contraindications, 57–58, 139
    dosage, 58–59, 60
    duration of action, 54, 55, 58
    effect on aura, 51
    efficacy, 52
    migraine abortion, 37, 44–52, 54, 55, 58, 59
Sunlight, as trigger factor, 113, 121
Superficial temporal artery, vasodilation, 10
Sympathetic nervous system, 7, 18
Sympathomimetic vasoconstrictors, 36–37
Symptomatic migraine, 23, 25

Synflex *See also* Naproxen sodium
  migraine abortion, 32, 34–35
  migraine prevention, 66, 81

Teichopsia *See* Scintillating scotoma
Tenormin, 66, 72 *See also* Atenolol
Tension-type vascular headache, 23–24
Thiethylperazine, 28
Thorazine, 28 *See also* Chlorpromazine
Tigan, 28 *See also* Trimethobenzamide
Timolol
  dosage, 97
  comparison with propranolol, 78
  efficacy, 75, 95
  migraine prevention, 66, 70, 78, 100
  mode of action, 101
Tolfenamic acid
  combination with caffeine, 35
  combination with metoclopramide, 35
  comparison with ergotamine, 35
  migraine abortion, 32, 35, 53
  migraine prevention, 80, 83
Torecan, 28 *See also* Thiethylperazine
Transient ischemic attacks, differentiating from migraine, 21
Traveling, as trigger factor, 121–122
Trazodone, childhood migraine, 123–127
Tricyclic antidepressants, 79–80, 95
Trigger factors, 2, 105
  aspartame, 115
  beer, 114
  caffeine, 115
  cheese, 114–115
  chocolate, 114
  citrus fruits, 114, 115
  cluster headache, 135–136
  estrogen cycle, 2, 105–110
  estrogen therapy, 111
  exercise, 121
  fluorescent lights, 121
  food additives, 115
  foods, 111, 114–115, 121, 122
  lack of sleep, 115, 122
  light, 122
  menopausal estrogen therapy, 111
  menstrual cycle, 2, 105–110
  monosodium glutamate, 115
  oral contraceptives, 110
  red wine, 114

  sleep, 115
  stress, 105, 111–112, 122
  sunlight, 113, 121
  traveling, 121–122
  weather changes, 111, 112–113, 121
Trimethobenzamide, 28
Tryptizol, 66, 78 *See also* Amitriptyline
Tyramine, as trigger factor, 114–115

Valium, 31 *See also* Diazepam
Valproate
  adverse effects, 96, 98
  contraindications, 99
  dosage, 98–99
  efficacy, 91, 95
  migraine prevention, 66, 89, 92–93, 100
  mode of action, 101
Vascular headache, 2–3
  cluster headache, 2, 22, 131–140
  tension-type, 23–24
Vasoconstrictor medications
  cluster headache, 133
  efficacy, 52–53
  migraine, 28, 29, 36–59
  rebound cycle, 55
Vasodilation, migraine pathogenesis, 9–10, 12–13, 15–18, 114–115
Vasodilators, 12, 14, 114–115
Verapamil
  adverse effects, 96, 98
  cluster headache, 138–139, 140
  contraindications, 98
  dosage, 98
  efficacy, 95
  migraine prevention, 66, 83, 87–89, 100
  mode of action, 100
  paroxysmal hemicrania, 140
Vistaril, 28 *See also* Hydroxyzine
Volatrol, 31–33 *See also* Diclofenac
Voltaren, 31–33 *See also* Diclofenac
Vomiting
  childhood migraine, 119, 121
  migraine, 4, 7, 23
  treatment, 27–28, 123

Weather changes, as trigger factor, 111, 112–113, 121
Wine, as trigger factor, 114